American Psychiatric Glossary

American Psychiatric Glossary

Compiled and Edited by

Evelyn M. Stone

Director, Facility for Continuing Medical Education
Director, Scientific Publications
McLean Hospital

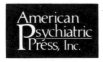

American Psychiatric Press, Inc.

**1400 K Street, N.W.
Washington, DC 20005**

Printing History
First Edition—1957, 265,000 copies
Second Edition—1964, 400,000 copies
Third Edition—1969, 450,000 copies
Fourth Edition—1975, 575,000 copies
Fifth Edition—1980, 400,000 copies
Sixth Edition—1988, 20,000 copies

88 89 90 91 8 7 6 5 4 3 2 1

Library of Congress Cataloging in Publication Data

Stone, Evelyn M.
    American psychiatric glossary.

    Rev. ed. of: The American Psychiatric Association's
psychiatric glossary. Trade ed. c1984.
    Bibliography: p.
    1. Psychiatry—Dictionaries.   I. American Psychiatric
Association's psychiatric glossary.   II. Title.   [DNLM:
1. Psychiatry-dictionaries.   WM 13 S8773a
RC437.S761   1988   616.89'003'21   87–26972
ISBN 0–88048–288–5

CONTENTS

INTRODUCTION AND ACKNOWLEDGMENTS

The vocabulary used in a scientific field undergoes continual change and refinement. Especially in a dynamic, clinical science such as psychiatry, definitions are modified to take into account new information about illness and recent developments in research. As more becomes known, the use of language becomes more precise, as does the application of diagnostic criteria. At times, change gives the false impression that illnesses are created or syndromes eliminated, whereas the process is actually one of redefinition. Since a glossary serves to define the words used in a particular field, *The American Psychiatric Glossary* undergoes periodic revision to keep its users abreast of current terminology.

This glossary incorporates the revised nomenclature of the American Psychiatric Association's new *Diagnostic and Statistical Manual (DSM-III-R)*. Diagnostic terms have been arranged and cross-referenced to allow easy use of the glossary by those familiar with the older nomenclature.

Words appearing in italics within a definition are defined elsewhere in the glossary, allowing convenient cross-checking. At times, the italicized word is listed alphabetically in a closely related form. For example, "psychotic" is not listed but *psychosis* is. In the tables, words that appear in boldface are defined elsewhere in the table or in the alphabetic listing in the glossary.

The construction "he or she" is a clumsy one to use in a glossary where brevity is essential. Therefore, we are using the conventional "he" when referring to a person of undesignated sex.

We were helped in producing the current glossary and the previous edition by the contributions of many experts in psychiatry and related fields. We are indebted to them all. Particular thanks are due to Martin Orne, MD, PhD, for the *Table of Research Terms*; to Steven Mirin, MD, and Roger Weiss, MD, for the *Table of Commonly Abused Drugs*; and to Ross Baldessarini, MD, for the current *Table of Drugs Used in Psychiatry*. I wish to thank also the distinguished editorial review panel for their diligence and support. I wish especially to thank Robert J. Campbell, M.D., for his skillful and always thoughtful editing of this editor's entries and definitions.

Other scholars who contributed various definitions and invaluable advice include: Scott Aaronson, MD, Richard I. Altesman, MD, Leona Bachrach, PhD, Walter E. Barton, MD, Arnold S. Berkman, PhD, Claire F. Berkman, EdD, Allan Beigel, MD, Thomas C. Bond, MD, Robert N. Butler, MD, Enoch Callaway, MD, Linn Campbell, MD, Pietro Castelnuovo-Tedesco, MD, Ronald Chen, MD, Bruce Cohen, MD, PhD, Jonathan O. Cole, MD, Stanley R. Dean, MD, John Donnelly, MD, Nancy A. Durant, MD, Norbert Enzer, MD, Aristide Esser, MD, Horacio Fabrega, Jr., MD, Fred M. Frankel, MD, Donald N. Haupt, MD, Barbara Herrington, Ernest R. Hilgard, PhD, Edward M. Hundert, MD, Phillip L. Isenberg, MD, Richard R. Kilburg, PhD, Joel Klein, Esq, Henry Krystal, MD, Alan Levenson, MD, Don R. Lipsitt, MD, Carolyn Maltas, PhD, Judd Marmor, MD, Steven Matthysse, PhD, A. Louis McGarry, MD, Harold McPheeters, MD, Lea Mesner, Sam Muszynski, Robert R. Nunn, MD, William Offenkrantz, MD, Lucy Ozarin, MD, Louis Paul, MD, Suzanne Quick, PhD, Edward Ritvo, MD, John Romano, MD, Lionel Rosen, MD, Arthur Rosenberg, Esq, Alan F. Schatzberg, MD, John M. Schneider, PhD, Victor Shashoua, PhD, Ronald Simons, MD, Robert Spitzer, MD, Thomas Stachnik, PhD, Irene Stiver, PhD, Samuel I. Stone, PhD, George E. Vaillant, MD, Lawrence Van Egeren, PhD, Marilyn Verhey, RN, Charles E. Wells MD, Arnold Werner, MD, Janet B. Williams, DSW, Robert L. Williams, MD, Bryan T. Woods, MD, Henry H. Work, MD.

For her patience typing and retyping many revisions, Carol Brown also deserves special thanks.

Evelyn M. Stone

A

abnormal In psychological terms, any mental or behavioral activity that deviates from culturally or scientifically determined norms.

abreaction Emotional release or discharge after recalling a painful experience that has been repressed because it was *consciously* intolerable. A therapeutic effect sometimes occurs through partial discharge or desensitization of the painful emotions and increased insight.

abstinence Voluntarily denying oneself some kind of gratification; in the area of alcohol or drug dependence, being without the substance on which the subject is dependent. The abstinence syndrome is equivalent to *withdrawal symptoms* and its appearance suggests the presence of physiologic dependence or *addiction*.

abstract attitude (categorical attitude) Cognitive functioning that includes assuming a mental set voluntarily; shifting voluntarily from one aspect of a situation to another, keeping in mind simultaneously various aspects of a situation; grasping the essentials of a whole, breaking it into its parts and isolating them voluntarily; planning ahead ideationally; and/or thinking or performing symbolically. A characteristic of many psychiatric disorders is the inability to assume the abstract attitude or to shift readily from the concrete to the abstract and back again as demanded by circumstances.

abulia Lack of will or motivation, often expressed as inability to make decisions. See *Table of Neurologic Deficits*.

abuse (child, elder, sexual, spouse) To misuse, attack, or injure. The most common form of abuse is child abuse. See *abused child*.

abused child A child or infant who has suffered repeated injuries, which may include bone fractures, neurologic and psychologic damage, and sexual abuse at the hands of a parent, parents, or parent surrogates. The abuse takes place repeatedly and is often precipitated, in the case of physical abuse, by the child's minor and normally irritating behavior. Child abuse also includes child neglect.

acalculia See *Table of Neurologic Deficits*.

accident-proneness Susceptibility to accidents based on psychologic causes or motivations.

accreditation A process by which hospitals and health facilities are surveyed and approved by the *Joint Commission on Accreditation of Hospitals* as measured against standards set by the commission.

acetylcholine One of the chemical neurotransmitters normally present in many parts of the body that enables nerve cells to signal each other.

acrophobia See *phobia*.

acting out Expressions of *unconscious* emotional conflicts or feelings in actions rather than words. The person is not *consciously* aware of the meaning of such acts. Acting out may be harmful or, in controlled situations, therapeutic (e.g. children's play therapy). Refers especially to acting out of *transference* wishes and emotions.

actualization Realization of one's full potential.

acute confusional state (1) A form of delirium in which the most prominent symptoms are disorders of memory and orientation, usually with short-term memory deficit and both retrograde and anterograde amnesia and clouding of consciousness (reduced clarity of awareness of environment with reduced capacity to shift, focus, and sustain attention to environmental stimuli). See *organic mental disorder*.
(2) An acute stress reaction, common in adolescence, to new surroundings or new demands; it generally subsides as the person adjusts to his situation. See also *identity crisis*.

adaptation Fitting one's behavior to meet the needs of one's environment which often involves a modification of one's impulses, emotions, or attitudes.

addiction Dependence on a chemical substance to the extent that a physiologic and/or psychologic need is established. This may be manifested by any combination of the following symptoms: tolerance, preoccupation with obtaining and using the substance, use of the substance despite anticipation of probable adverse consequences, repeated efforts to cut down or control substance use, and withdrawal symptoms when the substance is unavailable or not used.

adjustment Functional, often transitory, alteration or accommodation by which one can better adapt oneself to the immediate environment and to one's inner self. See also *adaptation*.

adjustment disorder A *DSM-III-R* category for maladaptive reactions to identifiable life events or circumstances. The symptoms generally lessen as the stress diminishes or as the person adapts to the stress.

Adler, Alfred (1870-1937) Viennese *psychiatrist,* founder of the school of *individual psychology. See also compensation, overcompensation,* and *masculine protest.*

administrative psychiatry The branch of psychiatry that deals with the organization of the efforts of many people in clinical practice, in a program, or in a hospital or other facility, to provide care and treatment. Its focus is on the management process formed by the interaction of health administration, clinical care of psychiatric patients, program elements, and the mental health organization itself with the attitudes, values, and belief systems of the environment in which the structure exists.

adolescence A chronologic period of growth beginning with physical and emotional processes leading to sexual and psychologic maturity at about age 12 and ending at a loosely defined time, when the individual achieves independence and social productivity (usually about age 20). This period is associated with rapid physical, psychologic, and social changes. See also *psychosocial development* and *psychosexual development.*

adrenergic Referring to neural activation by *catecholamines* such as *epinephrine, norepinephrine,* and *dopamine. See also sympathetic nervous system, biogenic amines,* and *neurotransmitters.*

adrenergic system That system of organs and nerves in which epinephrine (adrenalin) is the neurotransmitter.

adverse effects See *side effects.*

affect Subjective experience of emotion accompanying an idea or mental representation. The word affect is often used loosely as a generic term for feeling, emotion, or mood. Affect and *emotion* are commonly used interchangeably.

affect, flat Absence or near absence of any signs of affective expression.

affective disorder Disorder in which mood change or disturbance is the primary manifestation. See *depression*.

aftercare Posthospitalization program of rehabilitation designed to reinforce the effects of therapy and to help the patient adjust to his environment.

aggression Forceful physical, verbal, or symbolic action. May be appropriate and self-protective, including healthy self-assertiveness, or inappropriate as in hostile or destructive behavior. May also be directed toward the environment, toward another person or *personality*, or toward the self, as in *depression*.

aging Characteristic pattern of life changes that occur normally in humans, plants, and animals as they grow older. Some age changes begin at birth and continue until death; other changes begin at maturity and end at death.

agism Systematic stereotyping of and discrimination against elderly people to create distance from their social plight and to avoid primitive fears of aging and death. It is distinguished from gerontophobia, a specific pathologic fear of old people and aging.

6

agitated depression A severe major depressive disorder in which psychomotor agitation is prominent; formerly known as *involutional melancholia*. See *depression*.

agitation Excessive motor activity, usually nonpurposeful and associated with internal tension. Examples: inability to sit still, fidgeting, pacing, wringing of hands, or pulling of clothes.

agnosia Inability to understand the impact or significance of sensory stimuli. See *Table of Neurologic Deficits*.

agonist In pharmacology, a substance that promotes a receptor-mediated biologic response (contrast with *antagonist*).

agoraphobia Commonly, fear of leaving the familiar setting of one's home. In *DSM-III-R*, it is almost always a form of *panic disorder* rather than a *phobia*.

AIDS Acquired immune deficiency syndrome; a cluster of disorders such as Kaposi's sarcoma (KS) and opportunistic infections to which the subject is abnormally vulnerable because of collapse of the immune defense system. The cause is a retrovirus, human T-lymphocytic virus type III (HTLV-III) or HIV (human immunodeficiency virus), which infects and suppresses the T-4 lymphocyte, the focal cell of the immune system. It also directly attacks specific types of cells in the central nervous system and lungs (and perhaps in other tissues as well).

Approximately 70 percent of cases have occurred in homosexual and bisexual males, and about 25 percent in male and female intravenous drug users. There is no known cure and mortality rate is high.

Over 40 percent of AIDS patients develop neurologic complications at some point in their illness. The most common CNS dysfunction is a generalized encephalopathy or progressive multifocal leukoencephalopathy (PML) that includes dementia as a dominant feature. Less commonly, the dysfunction is due to well-defined focal lesions, including opportunistic infection by Toxoplasma gondii, which may invade nervous tissue and give rise to seizures or more subtle alterations in mentation and behavior. Cases with a presenting picture of acute psychosis without dementia have also been described. Myelopathy and peripheral neuropathy are other neurologic complications.

AIDS dementia characteristically begins with impaired concentration and mild memory loss and is often misdiagnosed as "reactive" depression or as a psychologic response to the threat of impending death. Over a period of several weeks or months the condition progresses to severe global cognitive impairment. Motor signs, including generalized hyperreflexia and increased tone, may accompany the dementia and some patients develop a spastic-ataxic gait or frank paraparesis. See *dementia*.

ailurophobia See *phobia*.

akathisia Motor restlessness ranging from a feeling of inner disquiet, often localized in the muscles, to inability to sit still or lie quietly; a side effect of some *antipsychotic drugs*. See also *Table of Neurologic Deficits*.

akinesia A state of motor inhibition; reduced voluntary movement. See also *Table of Neurologic Deficits*.

akinetic mutism See *Table of Neurologic Deficits*.

Al-Anon An organization of relatives of alcoholics operating in many communities under the philosophic and organizational structure of *Alcoholics Anonymous* to facilitate discussion and resolution of common problems.

Alateen An organization of teen-aged children of alcoholic parents operating in some communities under the philosophic and organizational structure of *Alcoholics Anonymous*. It provides a setting in which the children may receive group support in achieving a better understanding of their parents' problems and better methods for coping with them.

alcohol dependence (alcoholism) Dependence on alcohol characterized by either tolerance to the agent or development of *withdrawal* phenomena on cessation of, or reduction in, intake. Other aspects of the syndrome are psychologic dependence and impairment in social or vocational functioning. Medical complications include memory loss and liver dysfunction. See also *drug dependence*.

Alcohol, Drug Abuse, and Mental Health Administration (ADAMHA) An agency in the U.S. Department of Health and Human Services that provides leadership, policies, and goals for the federal effort to assure the treatment and rehabilitation of persons with alcohol abuse, *drug abuse*, and mental illness. ADAMHA is responsible for administering grants to advance and support research, and training, to individuals, institutions and agencies, and service programs through block grants to the states.

National Institute on Alcohol Abuse and Alcoholism (NIAAA) An institute within ADAMHA responsible for programs for the prevention, control, and research into courses and treatment of alcohol abuse and *alcoholism* and the rehabilitation of affected individuals.

National Institute on Drug Abuse (NIDA) An institute within ADAMHA responsible for the prevention, control, and research into causes and treatment of narcotic addiction and *drug dependence*.

National Institute of Mental Health (NIMH) An institute within ADAMHA responsible for programs dealing with *mental health*. The mission of NIMH is to improve the understanding, treatment and rehabilitation of the mentally ill, to prevent mental illness, and to foster the mental health of the American people. These goals are accomplished by supporting research, generating and transmitting new knowledge, demonstrating new technologies, and guiding national policy.

alcohol withdrawal syndrome See *delirium tremens*.

alcoholic hallucinosis An organic mental disorder consisting of auditory hallucinations occurring in a clear *sensorium*, developing shortly after the reduction or cessation of drinking, usually within 48 hours. It commonly follows prolonged and heavy alcohol use.

alcoholic psychoses A group of major *mental disorders* associated with organic brain damage due to alcohol; in *DSM-III-R* categorized as alcohol-induced organic mental disorders. Includes *delirium tremens*, *Wernicke-Korsakoff syndrome*, and *alcoholic hallucinosis*.

Alcoholics Anonymous (AA) A group of abstinent alcoholics who collectively assist other alcoholics through a structured program and personal and group support. *See also Al-Anon* and *Alateen*.

alcoholism A chronic illness manifested by repeated drinking that produces injury to one's health or to social or economic functioning.

Alexander, Franz (1891-1964) Hungarian *psychoanalyst*, professor of *psychoanalysis* at The University of Chicago; chief contributions were in areas of brief analytic and *psychosomatic* medicine.

alexia Loss of the power to grasp the meaning of written or printed words and sentences. *See Table of Neurologic Deficits. See also dyslexia.*

alexithymia A disturbance in affective and cognitive function which overlaps diagnostic entities but is common in *psychosomatic*, addictive, and *post-traumatic stress disorders*. The chief manifestation is difficulty in describing or recognizing one's own emotions, with a limited fantasy life and general constriction in the affective life.

algophobia Fear of pain. *See phobia.*

alienation The estrangement felt in a cultural setting one views as foreign, unpredictable, or unacceptable. For example, in *depersonalization* phenomena, feelings of unreality or strangeness produce a sense of alienation from one's self or environment. In obsessions, where there is fear of one's *emotions*, avoidance of situations that arouse emotions, and continuing effort to keep feelings out of awareness, there is alienation of *affect*.

alienist Obsolete term for a *psychiatrist* who testifies in court about a person's sanity or mental competence. See also *Table of Legal Terms*.

allied health professional A person with special training, working under the supervision of a health professional with responsibilities bearing on patient care.

alloplastic See *adaptation*.

Alzheimer's disease In *DSM-III-R*, primary degenerative *dementia* of the Alzheimer type; a degenerative organic mental disease with diffuse brain deterioration and progressive *dementia*. The symptoms are similar to *Pick's disease*. See also *senile dementia*, Alzheimer's type.

ambivalence The coexistence of contradictory *emotions*, attitudes, ideas, or desires with respect to a particular person, object, or situation. Ordinarily, it is not fully conscious and suggests psychopathology only when present in an extreme form.

amentia Subnormal development of the mind, with particular reference to intellectual capacities.

American Board of Psychiatry and Neurology (ABPN) A group of sixteen physicians (five from the *American Psychiatric Association*, four from the American Neurological Association, three from the Section Council on Psychiatry of the American Medical Association, two from the American Academy of Neurology, and two from the Section Council on Neurology of the American Medical Association). This group arranges, controls, and conducts examinations to determine the competence of specialists in psychiatry, child psychiatry, neurology, and neurology with special competence in child neurology.

American Journal of Psychiatry The official monthly scientific publication of the *American Psychiatric Association*.

American Law Institute formulation See *Table of Legal Terms*.

American Psychiatric Association (APA) The leading national professional organization in the United States for physicians who specialize in *psychiatry*. Members are from the United States, Canada, Central America, and the Caribbean Islands, and corresponding members from other countries. Founded in 1844 as the Association of Medical Superintendents of American Institutions for the Insane, the Association changed its name to the American Medico-Psychological Association in 1891 and adopted its present name in 1921. The Association is governed by a board of 19 elected trustees whose primary function is to formulate and implement the policies and programs of the Association, and by an Assembly of District Branches representing the membership which may approve or disapprove, but not reverse, actions of the Board of Trustees. Numerous councils, committees, commissions, and task forces furnish the data and recommendations on which the Trustees and Assembly base their deliberations. The Association had more than 33,000 members at the end of 1986. Its headquarters are at 1400 K Street, N.W., Washington, DC 20005.

amimia A disorder of language characterized by an inability to gesticulate or to understand the significance of gestures. See also *speech disturbances* and *learning disabilities*.

amines Organic compounds containing the amino group ($-NH_2$); of special importance in biochemistry and neurochemistry. See also *biologic psychiatry* and *biogenic amines.*

amino acids Any organic acid containing one or more amino ($-NH2_2$) groups. Amino acids are integral parts of proteins and are precursors of brain *neurotransmitters.*

amnesia Pathologic loss of memory; a phenomenon in which an area of experience becomes inaccessible to *conscious* recall. It may be organic, emotional, or of mixed origin, and limited to a sharply circumscribed period of time. Two types are:

> **retrograde** loss of memory for events preceding the amnesia proper and the condition(s) presumed to be responsible for it.

> **anterograde** inability to form new memories for events following such condition(s).

amok See *culture-specific syndromes.*

amphetamines A group of chemicals that stimulate the cerebral cortex of the brain; often misused by adults and adolescents to control normal fatigue and to induce euphoria. Used clinically to treat *hyperkinetic syndrome* and *narcolepsy.*

amygdala Part of the basal ganglia, located on the roof of the temporal horn of the lateral ventricle at the interior end of the caudate nucleus.

amyotrophic lateral sclerosis Motor *neuron* disease of unknown etiology characterized by progressive degeneration of cortico-spinal tracts and anterior horn cells or bulbar efferent neurons. Commonly known as "Lou Gehrig's disease."

anaclitic Literally, leaning on. In *psychoanalytic* terminology, dependence of the infant on the mother or mother substitute for a sense of well-being (e.g., gratification through nursing). Normal behavior in childhood, pathologic in later years if excessive.

anal character A *personality* type that manifests excessive orderliness, miserliness, and obstinacy. In *psychoanalysis*, a pattern of behavior in an adult that is believed to originate in the *anal phase* of infancy, between one and three years. See also *psychosexual development*.

anal phase See *psychosexual development*.

analgesia Absence of appreciation of painful sensations.

analysand A patient in *psychoanalytic* treatment.

analysis A common synonym for *psychoanalysis*.

analytic psychology The name given by the Swiss *psychoanalyst* Carl Gustav *Jung* to his theoretical system, which minimizes the influences of sexual factors in emotional disorders and stresses mystical religious influences and a belief in the collective unconscious.

anamnesis The developmental history of a patient and of his illness, especially his recollections.

anankastic personality Synonym for *obsessive compulsive* personality. See *compulsive personality* under *personality disorders*.

ancillary care Health services other than professional services, or hospital room and board; these services may include drug, laboratory, and therapy services.

androgyny A combination of male and female characteristics in one person.

anesthesia Absence of sensation; may result from nerve damage, anesthetic drugs, or psychologic processes such as in *hysterical neurosis, conversion type* (see under *neurosis*), or *hypnosis.*

anhedonia Inability to experience pleasure from activities that usually produce pleasurable feelings. Contrast with *hedonism.*

anima In Jungian psychology, a person's inner being as opposed to the character or *persona* presented to the world. Further, the anima may be the more feminine "soul" or inner self of a man; the animus the more masculine soul of a woman. See also *Jung.*

anniversary reaction An emotional response to a previous event occurring at the same time of year. Often the event involved a loss and the reaction involves a *depressed* state. The reaction can range from mild to severe and may occur at any time after the event.

anomie Apathy, alienation, and personal distress resulting from the loss of goals previously valued. Durkheim popularized this term when he listed it as a principal reason for suicide.

anorexia nervosa A disorder marked by severe and prolonged refusal to eat, with severe weight loss, amenorrhea or *impotence,* disturbance of body image, and an intense fear of becoming obese. Most frequently encountered in girls and young women. May be associated with *bulimia*.

anorgasmia The inability to achieve orgasm.

anosognosia See *Table of Neurologic Deficits*.

Antabuse (disulfiram) A drug used in treatment of *alcoholism* to create an aversive response to alcohol. It blocks the normal metabolism of alcohol and produces increased blood concentrations of acetaldehyde which cause very unpleasant reactions including flushing of the skin, pounding of the heart, shortness of breath, nausea, and vomiting. With more severe reactions, hypotension, cardiovascular collapse, and, sometimes, convulsions may occur.

antagonist A drug that reduces or blocks the action of another drug. For example, *naloxone* blocks the action of morphine by competing with it for receptor sites in the brain and other tissues. By occupying these sites, naloxone prevents the narcotic from binding to the receptors and exerting its effect. Contrast with *agonist*.

antianxiety drugs See *Table of Drugs Used in Psychiatry*.

anticholinergic effects or properties Interference with the action of acetylcholine in the brain and peripheral nervous systems by any drug. In *psychiatry*, the term generally refers to the side effects of *antipsychotic drugs*, *tricyclic antidepressants*, and *antiparkinson drugs*. Common symptoms of such effects include dry mouth, blurred vision, and constipation.

antidepressant drugs See *Table of Drugs Used in Psychiatry*.

antimanic drugs See *Table of Drugs Used in Psychiatry*.

antiparkinson drugs Pharmacologic agents that ameliorate Parkinson-like *symptoms*. In *psychiatry*, these agents are used to combat the untoward Parkinson-like and *extrapyramidal* effects that may be associated with treatment with phenothiazines and other antipsychotic drugs.

antipsychotic drugs See *Table of Drugs Used in Psychiatry*.

antisocial personality See *personality disorders*.

anxiety Apprehension, tension, or uneasiness from anticipation of danger, the source of which is largely unknown or unrecognized. Primarily of intrapsychic origin, in distinction to *fear*, which is the emotional response to a *consciously* recognized and usually external threat or danger. May be regarded as pathologic when it interferes with effectiveness in living, achievement of desired goals or satisfaction, or reasonable emotional comfort.

anxiety disorder A disorder in which *anxiety* is the most prominent feature. *DSM-III-R* classifies anxiety disorders as follows:
    panic disorder
        with agoraphobia
        without agoraphobia
    agoraphobia without history of panic disorder
    social phobia
    simple phobia
    obsessive compulsive disorder
    post-traumatic stress disorder
    generalized anxiety disorder

anxiety hysteria An early *psychoanalytic* term for what is now called *phobic neurosis* (see under *neurosis*).

anxiety neurosis See under *neurosis*.

anxiolytics Drugs that have an anti-anxiety effect and are used widely to relieve emotional tension. The most commonly used anti-anxiety drugs are the *benzodiazepines*. See *Table of Drugs Used in Psychiatry*.

apathy Lack of feeling, emotion, interest, or concern.

aphasia Loss of the ability to use or understand words. See *Table of Neurologic Deficits*.

aphonia Inability to produce normal speech sounds. May be due to either organic or psychologic causes.

apoplexy See *stroke*.

apperception Perception as modified and enhanced by one's own *emotions*, memories, and biases.

apraxia See *Table of Neurologic Deficits*.

arteriosclerosis See *cerebral arteriosclerosis*

artificial intelligence The study of *intelligence* using ideas and methods of computation whose central goal is to understand the principles that make intelligence possible.

assertiveness training A procedure in which subjects are taught appropriate interpersonal responses involving frank, honest, and direct expression of their feelings, both positive and negative.

assimilation A *Piagetian* term describing a person's ability to comprehend and integrate new experiences.

association Relationship between ideas and emotions by contiguity, continuity, or similarity. See also *free association* and *mental status*.

astereognosis See *Table of Neurologic Deficits*.

ataxia See *Table of Neurologic Deficits*.

attachment The behavior of an organism that relates in an affiliative or dependent manner to another object. This attachment develops during critical periods of life and can be extinguished by lack of opportunity to relate. If this separation occurs before maturation can provide for adaptive adjustment, personality deviation can occur.

attachment learning The theory that the presence of someone to whom we are emotionally attached has a special effect on how we learn, especially in infancy.

attention deficit disorder (ADD) A *DSM-III-R* category for a childhood disorder characterized by developmentally inappropriate short attention span, poor concentration, and frequent hyperactivity.

atypical An adjective used to describe unusual or uncharacteristic variations of a disorder.

atypical psychosis In *DSM-III-R*, a residual category for persons who have psychotic symptoms that do not meet the criteria for specific mental disorders. See also *psychosis*.

audit (medical audit, patient care audit) Periodic and systematic review of patterns of patient care to assess the quality of treatment.

aura A premonitory, subjective brief sensation (e.g., a flash of light) that warns of an impending headache or convulsion. The nature of the sensation depends on the brain area in which the attack begins. Seen in *migraine* and *epilepsy*.

authority figure A projected or real person in a position of power, e.g., a projected parent.

autism A pervasive developmental disorder caused by a physical disorder of the brain appearing during the first three years of life. Symptoms include disturbances in physical, social, and language skills; abnormal responses to sensations; and abnormal ways of relating to people, objects, and events.

autoeroticism Sensual self-gratification. Characteristic of, but not limited to, an early stage of emotional development. Includes satisfactions derived from genital play, masturbation, fantasy, and from oral, anal, and visual sources.

automatism Automatic and apparently undirected nonpurposive behavior that is not *consciously* controlled. Seen in psychomotor *epilepsy*.

autonomic nervous system (ANS) The part of the nervous system that innervates the cardiovascular, digestive, reproductive, and respiratory organs. It operates outside of consciousness and controls basic life-sustaining functions such as heart rate, digestion, and breathing. It includes the *sympathetic nervous system* and the *parasympathetic nervous system*.

autoplastic See *adaptation.*

autopsy, psychologic See *psychologic autopsy.*

aversion therapy A *behavior therapy* procedure in which stimuli associated with undesirable behavior are paired with a painful or unpleasant stimulus, resulting in the suppression of the undesirable behavior.

axon The long-nerve cell process that conducts impulses from the cell body.

B

barbiturates Drugs that depress the activities of the *central nervous system*; primarily used for sedation or treatment of convulsive disorders. See also *Table of Drugs Used in Psychiatry.*

basal ganglia Masses of grey matter lying deep within each cerebral hemisphere.

basic benefits In insurance policies, the minimum set of benefits which must be or are available to patients.

battered child See *abused child.*

beam See *brain electrical activity mapping.*

Beers, Clifford W. (1876-1943) Author of "A Mind That Found Itself" and founder, in 1909, of the National

Committee for Mental Hygiene, now the *National Mental Health Association*.

behavior disorders of childhood A group of behavior patterns occurring in childhood and *adolescence* that are less severe than *psychoses* but more resistant to treatment than transient situational disturbances because they are more stabilized and internalized. They are characterized by overactivity, inattentiveness, shyness, feelings of rejection, overaggressiveness, timidity, or delinquency. The child who frequently runs away from home or who persistently lies, steals, and teases other children in a hostile fashion falls into this category.

behavior modification See *behavior therapy*.

behavior therapy A mode of treatment that focuses on modifying observable and, at least in principle, quantifiable behavior by means of systematic manipulation of the environment and behavioral variables thought to be functionally related to the behavior. Some behavior therapy techniques are *operant conditioning, shaping, token economy, systematic desensitization, aversion therapy*, and *flooding*. Also see *biofeedback*.

behavioral neurology The branch of neurology that concerns itself with functioning, such as language, memory, and purposeful or motivated activity or *affect*.

behavioral sciences The study of human development, values, and interpersonal relations. The behavioral sciences encompass such fields as *psychiatry, psychology, cultural anthropology, sociology*, and political science.

behaviorism An approach to *psychology* first developed by *John B. Watson* which rejected the notion of mental states and reduced all psychologic phenomena to neural, muscular, and glandular responses. Contemporary behaviorism emphasizes the study of observable responses but is directed toward general behavior rather than discrete acts. It includes private events such as feelings and *fantasies* to the extent that these can be directly observed and measured.

benzodiazepines The generic name for a group of drugs that have potent hypnotic and sedative action. See also *Table of Drugs Used in Psychiatry*.

bereavement Feelings of deprivation, desolation, and grief at the loss of a loved one.

bestiality Zoophilia; sexual relations between a human being and an animal. See also *paraphilia*.

biochemistry The chemistry of living organisms and of the changes occurring therein.

biofeedback The use of instrumentation to provide information (feedback) about variations in one or more of the subject's own physiologic processes not ordinarily perceived, e.g. brainwave activity, muscle tension, or blood pressure. Such feedback over a period of time can help the subject learn to control certain physiologic processes even though he is unable to articulate how the learning was achieved.

biogenic amine hypothesis The concept that abnormalities in the physiology and metabolism of *biogenic amines*, particularly *catecholamines* (*norepinephrine* and *dopamine*) and an indoleamine (*serotonin*), are involved in the pathogenesis of certain psychiatric illnesses. The concept was derived originally from a serendipitous discovery that *monoamine oxidase inhibitors* and certain tricyclic drugs had mood-elevating properties, and that these agents exerted dramatic effect on brain monoamine functions. The findings that *phenothiazines* inhibit *dopamine* activity in the brain further support this theory and suggest that a disorder of dopamine metabolism may be implicated in the etiology of schizophrenia. Disorders in norepinephrine and serotonin activity have been implicated in the etiology of *depression* and *mania*.

biogenic amines Organic substances of interest because of their possible role in brain functioning. Subdivided into *catecholamines* (e.g., *epinephrine, dopamine, norepinephrine*) and *indoles* (e.g., tryptophan, *serotonin*).

biologic psychiatry A school of psychiatric thought that emphasizes physical, chemical, and neurologic causes of psychiatric illness and treatment approaches. See also *Table of Schools of Psychiatry*.

biologic rhythms Cyclical variations in physiologic and biochemical function, level of activity, and emotional state. Circadian rhythms have a cycle of about 24 hours; ultradian rhythms are shorter than one day; and infradian rhythms may be weeks or months.

bipolar 1 A disorder characterized by moderate to severe *hypomanic* or manic episodes requiring treatment or hospitalization for the excited state. These patients generally have recurrent episodes of *depression*.

bipolar 2 A disorder characterized by mild *hypomania* generally not requiring treatment. The patients may also have depressive episodes.

bipolar disorder A mood disorder in which there are episodes of both *mania* and *depression*; formerly called manic depressive psychosis, circular or mixed type. A mild form of bipolar disorder is sometimes labeled cyclothymic disorder. Bipolar disorder may be subdivided into manic, depressed, or mixed types on the basis of currently presenting *symptoms*.

manic Characterized by excitement, euphoria, expansive or irritable mood, hyperactivity, pressured speech, *flight of ideas*, decreased need for sleep, distractibility and impaired judgment. *Delusions* consistent with elation and grandiosity may be present.

depressed Characterized by lowered mood, slowed thinking, decreased movement or agitation, loss of interest, *guilt*, lowered self-esteem, *sleep* disturbance, decreased appetite, and ideas of suicide.

mixed Characterized by concomitant manic and depressive symptoms.

birth trauma Term used by *Rank* to relate his theories of *anxiety* and *neurosis* to what he believed to be the inevitable psychic shock of being born.

bisexuality Originally a concept of *Freud*, indicating a belief that components of both sexes could be found in each person. Today the term is often used to refer to persons who are capable of achieving *orgasm* with a partner of either sex. See also *gender role, homosexuality*.

Bleuler, Eugene (1857-1939) Swiss *psychiatrist* whose investigations of *dementia praecox* led him to outline a modern concept of *schizophrenia*.

blind spot An area of a person's personality of which he is totally unaware, since recognition would cause painful emotions.

blocking A sudden obstruction or interruption in spontaneous flow of thinking or speaking, perceived as an absence or deprivation of thought.

blood-brain barrier The barrier that excludes many molecules and substances from freely diffusing or being transported into the brain tissues from the blood stream; acts as a protective function.

blood levels The concentration of a drug in the plasma, serum, or blood. In *psychiatry*, the term is most often applied to levels of *lithium carbonate, tricyclic antidepressants*, and anticonvulsants. Maximum clinical responses to these agents have been correlated with specific ranges of blood levels. See also *therapeutic window*.

board-certified psychiatrist A *psychiatrist* who has passed examinations administered by the *American Board of Psychiatry and Neurology*, and thus becomes certified as a medical specialist in *psychiatry*.

board-eligible psychiatrist A *psychiatrist* who is eligible to take the examinations of the *American Board of Psychiatry and Neurology;* a psychiatrist who has completed an approved psychiatric residency training program.

body image One's sense of the self and one's body as presented to others.

body language The expression of feelings or thoughts transmitted by one's body motion, posture, or facial expressions that have meaning within the context in which they appear. See also *kinesics*.

bonding The attachment and unity of two people whose identities are significantly affected by their mutual interactions. Bonding often refers to the attachment between mother and her child.

borderline See under *personality disorders*.

bradykinetic syndrome Neurologic condition characterized by a generalized slowness of motor activity.

brain The part of the nervous system confined in the skull; it includes the cerebrum, midbrain, cerebellum, pons, and medulla.

brain disorders See *organic mental disorder*.

brain electrical activity mapping (BEAM) Computer-enhanced analysis and display of electroencephalographic and evoked response studies. In evoked response studies, a stimulus (e.g., flashing light) is presented to the patient and the responses are recorded electrically from scalp electrodes. Computers translate the information into a topographic, colored display of electrical activity over the surface of the brain. Useful in diagnosing seizure disorders and seems to be helpful in looking at atypical psychiatric presentations. See also *brain imaging*.

brain imaging Any technique that permits the in vivo visualization of the substance of the central nervous system. The best known of such techniques is *computerized axial tomography* (CT), commonly called the CAT scan. However, two newer methods of brain imaging, *positron-emission tomography* (PET) and *magnetic resonance imaging* (MRI), are based on different physical principles but also yield a series of two-dimensional images (or "slices") of brain regions of interest.

A number of other related techniques, such as ultrasound, angiography in its various forms, radionuclide scans, regional cerebral blood flow (RCBF) measurements, *brain electrical activity mapping* (BEAM) and its variants, and even the older pneumoencephalogram (PEG) also provide images of some aspect of the central nervous system, but are generally more limited in the structures visualized or degree of resolution, or some other parameter, than CT, PET, and MRI.

brain metabolism The process by which the brain synthesizes, degrades and alters its cells for repair and function.

brain stem The pons and the medulla oblongata.

brain syndrome See *organic mental disorder*.

brain waves See *electroencephalogram*.

Brawner decision See *American Law Institute Formulation* under *Table of Legal Terms*.

brief psychotherapy Any form of *psychotherapy*, the end point of which is defined either in terms of the number of sessions (generally not more than 15) or in terms of specified objectives; usually goal-oriented, circumscribed, active, focused, and directed toward a specific problem or *symptom*.

brief reactive psychosis A *DSM-III-R* category for a psychosis lasting less than one week, with sudden onset after major stress.

Brigham, Amariah (1798-1849) One of the original thirteen founders of the *American Psychiatric Associa-*

tion (1844) and the founder and first editor of its official journal, now the *American Journal of Psychiatry*.

Briquet's syndrome See *somatization disorder*.

bruxism Grinding of the teeth, occurs *unconsciously* while awake or during stage *2 sleep*. May be secondary to *anxiety*, tension, or dental problems.

bulimia Episodic eating binges or excessive intake of food or fluid, generally beyond voluntary control. Characteristics are self-induced vomiting and purging following eating, which is of the binge-eating variety. The resulting loss of body fluids and electrolytes may lead to severe disturbances such as EKG abnormalities and tetany. Sometimes seen as a *symptom* in *anorexia nervosa*.

burnout A stress reaction developing in persons working in an area of unrelenting occupational demands. *Symptoms* include impaired work performance, fatigue, *insomnia*, *depression*, increased susceptibility to physical illness, and reliance on alcohol or other drugs of abuse for temporary relief.

butyrophenones See *Table of Drugs Used in Psychiatry*.

C

cannabis See *Table of Commonly Abused Drugs*.

capitation A form of prospective payment based on the size of the population covered. The health-care provider or group of providers accepts responsibility to deliver the health services needed by all members of a specified group, and an agreed-upon payment is made at regular intervals to them. The payment is made even if no services have been given; but the payment is no greater than the agreed-upon amount even if very many services have been provided.

care and protection proceedings See *Table of Legal Terms.*

caregiver Any person involved in the identification or prevention of illness or in the treatment or rehabilitation of the patient; includes the psychiatrist and other members of the traditional treatment team as well as community workers and other non-professionals.

castration Removal of the sex organs. In psychologic terms, the fantasized loss of the genitals. Also used figuratively to denote state of *impotence*, powerlessness, helplessness, or defeat.

castration anxiety *Anxiety* due to fantasized danger or injuries to the genitals and/or body. May be precipitated by everyday events which have symbolic significance and appear to be threatening, such as loss of a job, loss of a tooth, or an experience of ridicule or humiliation.

CAT scan See *computerized axial tomography.*

catalepsy A generalized condition of diminished responsiveness usually characterized by trance–like states. May occur in organic or psychologic disorders, or under *hypnosis.*

catatonia Immobility with muscular rigidity or inflexibility and at times excitability. See also *schizophrenia*.

catchment area A geographic area for which a mental health program or facility has responsibility for its residents.

catecholamines A group of *biogenic amines* derived from phenylalanine and containing the catechol nucleus. Certain of these amines, such as *epinephrine*, *norepinephrine*, and *dopamine*, are neurotransmitters and exert an important influence on peripheral and *central nervous system* activity.

categorical attitude See *abstract attitude*.

catharsis The healthful (therapeutic) release of ideas through a "talking out" of *conscious* material accompanied by an appropriate emotional reaction. Also, the release into awareness of repressed (i.e., "forgotten") material from the *unconscious*. See also *repression*.

cathexis Attachment, *conscious* or *unconscious*, of emotional feeling and significance to an idea, an object, or most commonly a person.

causalgia A sensation of burning pain of either organic or psychologic origin. See also *somatoform disorder*.

central nervous system (CNS) The brain and the spinal cord.

cephalalgia Headache or head pain.

cerea flexibilitas The "waxy flexibility" often present in catatonic *schizophrenia* in which the patient's arm or leg remains in the position in which it is placed.

cerebral arteriosclerosis Hardening of the arteries of the brain sometimes resulting in an *organic mental disorder* that may be either primarily neurologic (e.g. convulsions, *aphasia*, chorea, athetosis, *parkinsonism*, etc.) or primarily psychologic (e.g. intellectual dulling, memory deficits, emotional *lability*, paranoid *delusions*, and confusion) or a combination of both.

cerebrovascular accident (CVA) See *stroke*.

character The sum of a person's relatively fixed *personality* traits and habitual modes of response.

character analysis *Psychoanalytic* treatment aimed at the character defenses.

character defense Any character or personality trait which serves an *unconscious* defensive purpose. See also *defense mechanism*.

character disorder (character neurosis) A personality disorder manifested by a chronic, habitual, maladaptive pattern of reaction that is relatively inflexible, limits the optimal use of potentialities, and often provokes the responses from the environment that the person wants to avoid. In contrast to symptoms of *neurosis*, character traits are typically *ego-syntonic*. See also *personality*.

child abuse See *abused child*.

child analysis Application of modified *psychoanalytic* methods and goals to problems of children to remove impediments to normal personality development.

childhood schizophrenia See *schizophrenia*.

chlorpromazine See *Table of Drugs Used in Psychiatry*.

cholinergic Activated or transmitted by acetylcholine (e.g. parasympathetic nerve fibers). See also *parasympathetic nervous system*. Contrast with *adrenergic*.

chromosome 21 The chromosome involved in *Down's syndrome* (21 trisomy) which is most frequently due to nondisjunction of chromosome 21, resulting in three, rather than two, chromosomes (and making the total 47 chromosomes, rather than the normal total of 46). In 1987, it was reported that the genetic defect in familial *Alzheimer's* is located on chromosome 21, the same chromosome of which there is an extra copy in Down's syndrome. This supports the idea that at least one form of Alzheimer's is inherited, and that a similar genetic defect may occur in both familial Alzheimer's and Down's syndromes.

chromosomes Microscopic, intranuclear structures that carry the *genes*. The normal human cell contains 46 chromosomes, consisting of 23 pairs of chromosomes—22 pairs of autosomes and one pair of sex chromosomes.

chronic Continuing over a long period of time or recurring frequently. Chronic conditions often begin inconspicuously and symptoms are less pronounced than in acute conditions.

chronobiology The science or study of temporal factors in life stages and disorders, such as the sleep-waking cycle, biologic clocks and rhythms, etc.

circadian rhythms See *biologic rhythms*.

circumstantiality Pattern of speech that is indirect and delayed in reaching its goal. Compare with *tangentiality*.

clanging A type of thinking in which the sound of a word, rather than its meaning, gives the direction to subsequent associations; punning and rhyming may substitute for logic, and language may become increasingly a senseless *compulsion* to associate and decreasingly a vehicle for communication.

claustrophobia See *phobia*.

climacteric Menopausal period in women. Sometimes used to refer to the corresponding age period in men.

clinical psychologist See *psychologist*.

cluster suicides Multiple suicides, usually among adolescents, in a circumscribed period of time and area. Thought to have an element of contagion.

CME See *continuing medical education*.

cocaine A naturally occurring stimulant drug found in the leaves of the coca plant *Erythroxylon coca*. Its systemic effects include nervous system stimulation, manifested by garrulousness, restlessness, excitement, delusional ideas, and a false feeling of increased strength and mental capacity.

cognition A general term encompassing all the various modes of knowing and reasoning.

cognitive Refers to the mental process of comprehension, judgment, memory, and reasoning, as contrasted with emotional and volitional processes. Contrast with *conative*.

cognitive development Beginning in infancy, the acquisition of intelligence, *conscious* thought, and problem-solving abilities. An orderly sequence in the increase in knowledge derived from sensorimotor activity has been empirically demonstrated by *Piaget*. See also *psychosexual development* and *psychosocial development*.

cognitive therapy A treatment method particularly for depressive disorders, that emphasizes the rearrangement of a person's maladaptive processes of thinking, perceptions, and attitudes.

collective unconscious In Jungian theory, a portion of the unconscious common to all people; also called "racial unconscious." See also *analytic psychology*, *Jung*, and *unconscious*.

coma An abnormal state of depressed responsiveness with absence of adaptational response to tactile, thermal, proprioceptive, visual, auditory, olfactory, or verbal stimuli. See also *organic mental disorder*.

combat fatigue Disabling physical and emotional reaction incident to military combat. Paradoxically, the reaction may not necessarily include fatigue; an outmoded term especially common in World War II, now replaced by *post-traumatic stress* disorder occurring as a result of military combat.

commitment A legal process for admitting a mentally ill person to a psychiatric treatment program. The legal definition and procedure vary from state to state although commitment usually requires a court or judicial procedure. Commitment may also be voluntary.

community mental health center (CMHC) A mental health service delivery system first authorized by the federal Mental Retardation Facilities and Community Mental Health Center Construction Act of 1963, to provide a comprehensive program of mental health care to *catchment area* residents. The CMHC is typically a community facility or a network of affiliated agencies that serves as a locus for the delivery of the various services included in the concept of *community psychiatry*. Current regulations governing federal support for the centers require that they offer at least 10 services: inpatient, outpatient, partial hospitalization, emergency services, consultation and education, specialized services for children and the elderly, transitional halfway house services, alcohol and drug abuse services, assistance to courts and other public agencies, and follow-up care.

community psychiatry That branch of *psychiatry* concerned with the provision and delivery of a coordinated program of mental health care to residents of a designated geographic area termed the *catchment area*.

compensation A *defense mechanism*, operating *unconsciously*, by which one attempts to make up for real or fancied deficiencies. Also a *conscious* process in which one strives to make up for real or imagined defects of physique, performance skills, or psychologic attributes. The two types frequently merge. See also *Adler, individual psychology*, and *overcompensation*.

compensation neurosis Factitious illness, complicated by unresolved monetary claims.

competency to stand trial see *Table of Legal Terms*.

complex A group of associated ideas having a common, strong emotional tone. These are largely *unconscious* and significantly influence attitudes and associations. See also *Oedipus complex*.

compulsion An insistent, repetitive, intrusive, and unwanted urge to perform an act that is contrary to one's ordinary wishes or standards. Since it serves as a defensive substitute for still more unacceptable *unconscious* ideas and wishes, failure to perform the compulsive act leads to overt *anxiety*.

compulsive personality See *personality disorder*.

computerized axial tomography (CAT scanning, CT) A technique for imaging anatomical structures using x-ray. Objects are exposed to a series of x-ray beams on a single plane but with origin at different points around a 180-degree arc. A computer algorithm reconstructs the beam absorption data so as to display an image of absorption values at each point in the plane. The process is repeated for each plane to be imaged. Used for anatomical abnormalities such as strokes, tumor, atrophy of the brain. See also *brain imaging*.

conative Pertains to one's basic strivings as expressed in behavior and actions; volitional as contrasted with *cognitive*.

concordance See *Table of Research Terms*.

concrete thinking Thinking characterized by immediate experience, rather than abstractions. Seen in persons who have never developed the ability to generalize.

concussion An impairment of brain function caused by injury to the head. The speed and degree of recovery depend on severity of the brain injury. *Symptoms* may include headache, disorientation, paralysis, and occasionally unconsciousness.

condensation A psychologic process often present in dreams in which two or more concepts are fused so that a single symbol represents the multiple components.

conditioning Establishing new behavior as a result of psychologic modifications of responses to stimuli.

conditioning, operant See *operant conditioning*.

conditioning, respondent See *respondent conditioning*.

confabulation See *Table of Neurologic Deficits*.

confidentiality The ethical principle that a physician may not reveal any information disclosed in the course of medical attendance. See also *privilege, privileged communication* in *Table of Legal Terms*.

conflict A mental struggle that arises from the simultaneous operation of opposing *impulses, drives,* external (environmental) or internal demands. Termed *intrapsychic* when the conflict is between forces within the personality; extrapsychic, when it is between the self and the environment.

confrontation A communication that deliberately invites another to self-examine some aspect of behavior in which there is a discrepancy between saying and doing.

confusion Disturbed orientation in respect to time, place, or person. See *delirium, dementia, mental status, organic mental disorder*.

congenital Literally, present at birth. It may include conditions that arise during fetal development or with the birth process as well as hereditary or genetically determined conditions. It does not refer to conditions that appear after birth.

conjoint therapy A form of *marital therapy* in which a therapist sees the partners together in joint sessions.

conscience The morally self-critical part of one's standards of behavior, performance, and value judgments. Commonly equated with the *superego*.

conscious The content of mind or mental functioning of which one is aware. In neurology, awake, alert. See also *unconscious*.

conservatorship See *Table of Legal Terms*.

constitution A person's intrinsic physical and psychologic endowment; sometimes used more narrowly to indicate physical inheritance or intellectual potential.

constitutional types Constellations of morphologic, physiologic, and psychologic traits as earlier proposed by various scholars. Galen: sanguine, melancholic, choleric, and phlegmatic types; Kretschmer: pyknic (stocky), asthenic (slender), athletic, and dysplastic (disproportioned) types; Sheldon: ectomorphic (thin), mesomorphic (muscular), and endomorphic (fat) types, based on the relative preponderance of outer, middle, or inner layers of embryonic cellular tissue.

consultation liaison psychiatry An area of special interest in general psychiatry which addresses the interpersonal, psychologic, and psychosocial aspects of all medical care, particularly in a general hospital setting. The liaison *psychiatrist* works closely with medical-surgical physicians and nonphysician staff to enhance the diagnosis, treatment, and management of the patient with illness considered primarily nonpsychiatric. Consultation may be to any part of the health care system which affects the patient and the family. It may occasionally lead to a recommendation or referral for more specific psychotherapy, but more typically consists of short-term intervention by a "liaison team" with a biopsychosocial approach to illness.

continuing medical education (CME) Postgraduate educational activities aimed at maintaining, updating, and extending professional knowledge and skills. Many professional organizations and state licensing boards require participation in CME activities.

contract Explicit commitment between patient and therapist to a well defined course of action to achieve the treatment goal.

control group See *Table of Research Terms*.

conversion A *defense mechanism*, operating *unconsciously*, by which *intrapsychic conflicts* that would otherwise give rise to *anxiety* are, instead, given symbolic external expression. The repressed ideas or impulses, and the psychologic defenses against them, are converted into a variety of somatic *symptoms* involving the nervous system. These may include such symptoms as paralysis, pain, or loss of sensory function.

conversion disorder *DSM-III-R* term for *hysterical neurosis, conversion type.* See under *neurosis.*

conviction A firm and settled belief.

convulsive disorders Primarily the centrencephalic seizures, grand mal and petit mal, and the focal seizures of Jacksonian and psychomotor *epilepsy.* These brain disorders, with their characteristic *electroencephalographic* patterns, are to be differentiated from a variety of other pathophysiologic conditions in which a convulsive seizure may occur. For example, such seizures may follow withdrawal from alcohol, *barbiturates,* and a wide variety of other drugs; they may also occur in cerebral vascular disease, brain tumor, brain abscess, *hypoglycemia,* hyponatremia, and many other metabolic and intracranial disorders.

coping mechanisms Ways of adjusting to environmental stress without altering one's goals or purposes; includes both *conscious* and *unconscious* mechanisms.

coprophagia Eating of filth or feces.

coprophilia Excessive or morbid interest in filth or feces or their symbolic representations.

correlation See *Table of Research Terms.*

counseling A therapeutic device of conversation and discussion in which one individual offers advice or guidance to another on particular or general personal problems. The method is commonly used by *psychiatrists, social workers,* and the clergy.

counterphobia The desire for seeking out experiences that are *consciously* or *unconsciously* feared.

countertransference The *psychiatrist's* partly *unconscious* or *conscious* emotional reactions to the patient. See also *transference*.

couples therapy See *marital therapy*.

crack Freebase or alkaloidal cocaine. See also *Table of Commonly Abused Drugs*.

cretinism A type of *mental retardation* and bodily malformation caused by severe, uncorrected thyroid deficiency in infancy and early childhood.

cri du chat Syndrome of *mental retardation*. The name is derived from a catlike cry emitted by children with this disorder, which is caused by partial deletion of the fifth chromosome.

criminal responsibility See *Table of Legal Terms*.

crisis A state of psychological disequilibrium; turning point in a person's life.

crisis intervention A form of *brief psychotherapy* that emphasizes identification of the specific event precipitating the emotional trauma and uses methods to neutralize that trauma. Often used in hospital emergency rooms.

cross-cultural psychiatry The comparative study of *mental illness* and *mental health* among different societies, nations, and cultures. Often used synonymously with transcultural psychiatry.

cross-dressing See *transvestism*.

cult A system of beliefs and rituals based on dogma or religious teachings.

cultural anthropology The study of man and his works or of the learned behavior of man: technology, languages, religions, values, customs, mores, beliefs, social relationships, and family life and structure. Similar to social anthropology and *ethnology*.

cultural psychiatry A branch of *social psychiatry* concerned with the mentally ill in relation to their cultural environment. *Symptoms* of behavior regarded as psychopathologic in one society may be regarded as acceptable and normal in another.

culture shock Feelings of isolation, rejection and alienation experienced by an individual or group when transplanted from a familiar to an unfamiliar culture, e.g., from one country to another.

culture-specific syndromes Forms of disturbed behavior specific to certain cultural systems that do not conform to western *nosologic* entities. commonly cited syndromes are

Syndrome	Culture	Symptoms
amok	Malay	acute indiscriminate homicidal mania
koro	Chinese, S.E. Asia	fear of retraction of penis into abdomen with the belief that this will lead to death
latah	S.E. Asia	startle-induced disorganization, hypersuggestibility, automatic obedience, and *echopraxia*.

| **piblokto** | Eskimo | attacks of screaming, crying, and running naked through the snow |
| **windigo** | Canadian Indians | *delusions* of being possessed by a cannabalistic monster (windigo), attacks of agitated *depression*, oral *sadistic* fears and impulses |

CVA (cerebro vascular accident). *See* stroke.

cyclothymic disorder A mild form of *bipolar disorder*.

D _____

Da Costa's syndrome Neurocirculatory asthenia; "soldier's heart."

day hospital See *partial hospitalization*.

day residue Any element of a dream that is clearly derived from some event of the previous day. The day residue is often useful in deciphering meaning from the dream.

death instinct (Thanatos) In Freudian theory, the *unconscious* drive toward dissolution and death. Coexists with and is in opposition to the life *instinct* (Eros).

decompensation The deterioration of existing *defenses*, leading to an exacerbation of pathologic behavior.

defense mechanism *Unconscious* intrapsychic processes serving to provide relief from emotional *conflict* and *anxiety*. *Conscious* efforts are frequently made for the same reasons, but true defense mechanisms are unconscious. Some of the common defense mechanisms defined in this glossary are: *compensation, conversion, denial, displacement, dissociation, idealization, identification, incorporation, introjection, projection, rationalization, reaction formation, regression, sublimation, substitution, symbolization,* and *undoing.*

deficit Insufficient quantity or inadequate supply. In neurology it refers to inability to perform (e.g., a motor action) because of some interference along the chain of neurophysiologic and neurochemical events that lies between stimulus and response.

deinstitutionalization Change in locus of mental health care from traditional, institutional settings to community-based services. Sometimes called transinstitutionalization because it often merely shifts the patients from one institution (the hospital) to another (such as a prison).

déjà vu A paramnesia consisting of the sensation or illusion that one is seeing what one has seen before.

delirium An acute *organic mental disorder* characterized by confusion and altered, possibly fluctuating, *consciousness* due to an alteration of cerebral metabolism; it may include *delusions, illusions,* and/or *hallucinations.* The condition is reversible if the underlying cause can be identified and treated. It may, however, progress to *dementia* or death. Often emotional *lability*, typically appearing as *anxiety* and *agitation*, is present. Contrast with *dementia*.

delirium tremens An acute and sometimes fatal brain disorder (in 10-15% of untreated cases) caused by total or partial withdrawal from excessive alcohol intake. Usually develops in 24-96 hours after cessation of drinking. *Symptoms* include fever, tremors, ataxia and sometimes convulsions, frightening *illusions*, *delusions*, and *hallucinations*. The condition is often accompanied by nutritional deficiencies. It is a medical emergency. Contrast with *alcoholic hallucinosis*. See also *Wernicke-Korsakoff syndrome*.

delusion A false belief firmly held despite incontrovertible and obvious proof or evidence to the contrary. Further, the belief is not one ordinarily accepted by other members of the person's culture or subculture. See also *delusional (paranoid) disorder*.

delusional depression Severe depressive disorder characterized by psychotic thinking (e.g. *delusions* or *hallucinations*) as well as neurovegetative symptoms. Listed in *DSM-III-R* as major depression, severe, with psychotic features.

delusional (paranoid) disorder A mental disorder characterized by a persistent mental disorder such as *schizophrenia*, *schizophreniform disorder*, *mood* disorder, or *organic mental* disorder. Auditory or visual hallucinations, if present, are not prominent. Delusional (paranoid) disorders are usually subtyped by the predominant delusional theme: erotomanic, grandiose, jealous, persecutory, or somatic.

dementia An *organic mental disorder* in which there is a deterioration of previously acquired intellectual abilities of sufficient severity to interfere with social or occupational functioning. Memory disturbance is the most prominent *symptom*. In addition, there is impairment of abstract thinking, judgment, impulse control, and/or personality change. Dementia may be progressive, static, or reversible, depending on the pathology and the availability of effective treatment. See also *senile dementia*. Contrast with *delirium*.

dementia praecox Obsolete descriptive term for *schizophrenia*. Introduced by Morel (1860) and later popularized by *Kraepelin*.

dementia, senile See *senile dementia*.

demography The study of a population and those variables bringing about change in that population. See also *epidemiology*.

dendrite A branch of the nerve cell that receives nerve impulses from the stem of a neighboring nerve.

denial A *defense mechanism*, operating *unconsciously*, used to resolve emotional *conflict* and allay *anxiety* by disavowing thoughts, feelings, wishes, needs, or external reality factors that are *consciously* intolerable.

deoxyribonucleic acid (DNA) Chemical substance found in chromosomes within cell nuclei; its molecular structure contains the organism's genetic information.

dependency needs Vital needs for mothering, love, affection, shelter, protection, security, food, and warmth. May be a manifestation of *regression* when they reappear openly in adults.

dependent personality disorder Disorder characterized by a lack of self-confidence, a tendency to have others assume responsibility for one's life, and subordination of one's needs and wishes to the person(s) on whom one is dependent.

depersonalization Feelings of unreality or strangeness concerning either the environment, the self, or both. See also *neurosis* and *derealization*.

depersonalization disorder (neurosis) *DSM-III-R* term for depersonalization *neurosis*. See *neurosis*.

depression When used to describe a *mood*, depression refers to feelings of sadness, despair and discouragement. As such, depression may be a normal feeling state. The overt manifestations are highly variable and may be *culture specific*. Depression may be a *symptom* seen in a variety of mental or physical disorders, a *syndrome* of associated symptoms secondary to an underlying disorder, or a specific *mental disorder*. Slowed thinking, decreased pleasure, decreased purposeful physical activity, *guilt* and hopelessness, and disorders of eating and sleeping may be commonly seen in the depressive syndrome. *DSM-III-R* classifies depression by severity, recurrence, and association with *hypomania* or *mania*.

Other categorizations divide depression into reactive and endogenous depressions on the basis of precipitants or symptom clusters. In *DSM-III-R*, an episode of the occurrence of an endogenous depressive symptoms cluster is generally referred to as a moderate or severe episode of a major depressive syndrome, melancholic type. In *DSM-II*, depression was referred to as *psychotic* when severe functional impairment occurred, but in *DSM-III-R*, psychosis refers to a *reality testing*, manifested by delusions or hallucinations. Depression in children may be manifested by refusal to go to school, *anxiety*, excessive reaction to separation from parental figures, antisocial behavior, and somatic complaints.

deprivation, emotional Lack of adequate and appropriate interpersonal and/or environmental experience, usually in the early developmental years.

deprivation, sensory See *sensory deprivation*.

depth psychology The psychology of *unconscious* mental processes. Also a system of *psychology* in which the study of such processes plays a major role, as in *psychoanalysis*.

derealization A feeling of detachment from one's environment. May be accompanied by *depersonalization*.

dereistic Mental activity that is not in accordance with reality, logic, or experience. See also *autism*.

descriptive psychiatry A system of *psychiatry* based on the study of readily observable external factors. Often used to refer to the systematized descriptions of mental illness formulated by *Kraepelin*. Contrast with *dynamic psychiatry*.

desensitization See *systematic desensitization*.

designer drugs Addictive drugs that are synthesized or manufactured to give the same subjective effects as well known illicit drugs. Since the process is a covert operation there is great difficulty in tracing the manufacturer to check the drugs for adverse effects.

detachment A behavior pattern characterized by general aloofness in interpersonal contact; may include intellectualization, denial, and superficiality.

determinism The theory that one's emotional life does not result from chance alone but rather from specific causes or forces, known or unknown.

detoxification Treatment by the use of medication, diet, rest, fluids, and nursing care to restore physiologic functioning after it has been seriously disturbed by the overuse of alcohol, *barbiturates*, or other *addictive* drugs.

developmental disorder A handicap or impairment originating before the age of 18 which may be expected to continue indefinitely and which constitutes a substantial impairment. The disability may be attributable to *mental retardation*, cerebral palsy, *epilepsy*, or other neurologic conditions and may include *autism*.

diagnosis The process of determining, through examination and analysis, the nature of a patient's illness.

Diagnostic and Statistical Manual of Mental Disorders (DSM)

DSM-I The first edition of the *American Psychiatric Association's* official classification of mental disorders, published in 1952.

DSM-II The second edition published in 1968.

DSM-III The third edition, published in 1980.

DSM-III-R The revised DSM-III, published in 1987.

diagnostic related groups (DRG) Classification representing 23 major diagnostic categories that aggregates patients into case types based on diagnosis. A diagnosis related group is a subset of a major diagnostic category.

differential diagnosis The consideration of which of two or more diseases with similar symptoms the patient suffers from.

differentiation The degree to which an individual identifies the self as separate or distinct from others.

disability (psychiatric) Deprivation of intellectual or emotional capacity or fitness. As defined by the federal government, "Inability to engage in any substantial gainful activity by reason of any medically determinable physical or mental impairment which can be expected to last or has lasted for a continuous period of not less than 12 full months." See also *developmental disability*.

disconnection syndrome Term coined by Norman Geschwind (1926-1984) to describe the interruption of information transferred from one brain region to another.

discordance See *Table of Research Terms*.

disinhibition Freedom to act according to one's inner drives or feelings, with less regard for restraints imposed by cultural norms or one's superego; removal of an inhibitory constraining, or limiting influence, as in the escape from higher cortical control in neurologic injury, or in uncontrolled firing of impulses when a drug interferes with the usual limiting or inhibiting action of *GABA* within the central nervous system.

disorientation Loss of awareness of the position of the self in relation to space, time, or other persons; confusion. See also *delirium* and *dementia*.

displacement A *defense mechanism*, operating *unconsciously*, in which emotions, ideas, or wishes are transferred from their original object to a more acceptable substitute; often used to allay *anxiety*.

dissociation The splitting off of clusters of mental contents from conscious awareness, a mechanism central to hysterical conversion and dissociative disorders; the separation of an idea from its emotional significance and affect as seen in the inappropriate *affect* of schizophrenic patients.

dissociative disorder Category of disorders in *DSM-III-R* in which there is a sudden, temporary alteration in normally integrated functions of *consciousness*, identity, or motor behavior, so that some part of one or more of these functions is lost. It includes psychogenic *amnesia*, psychogenic *fugue*, *multiple personality*, and *depersonalization disorder*.

distractibility Inability to maintain attention; shifting from one area or topic to another with minimal provocation. Distractibility may be a manifestation of organic impairment or it may be a part of a functional disorder such as *anxiety* states, *mania*, or *schizophrenia*.

distributive analysis and synthesis The therapy used by the psychobiologic school of psychiatry developed by *Meyer*; entails extensive guided and directed investigation and analysis of the patient's entire past experience, stressing assets and liabilities to make possible a constructive synthesis. See also *psychobiology*.

Dix, Dorothea Lynde (1802-1887) Foremost nineteenth-century American crusader for the improvement of institutional care of the mentally ill.

dizygotic twins Twins who develop from two separately fertilized ova. Also called fraternal twins.

DNA See *deoxyribonucleic acid.*

dominance A predisposition to play a prominent or controlling role when interacting with others. In *neurology,* the (normal) tendency of one-half of the brain to be more important than the other in mediating various functions (cerebral dominance). In genetics, the ability of one *gene* (dominant gene) to express itself in the *phenotype* of an individual, even though that gene is paired with another (recessive gene) that would have expressed itself in a different way.

dopamine A neurosynaptic transmitter found in the brain, specifically associated with some forms of *psychosis* and abnormal movement disorders. See also *biogenic amines.*

dopamine hypothesis A theory that attempts to explain the pathogenesis of *schizophrenia* and other psychotic states as due to excesses in *dopamine* activity in various areas of the brain. This theory is, in part, based on biologic observations that the antipsychotic properties of specific drugs may be related to their ability to block the action of dopamine.

double bind Interaction in which one person demands a response to a message containing mutually contradictory signals, while the other person is unable either to comment on the incongruity or to escape from the situation.

double blind See *Table of Research Terms.*

double personality See *multiple personality.*

Down's syndrome Also known as trisomy 21, a common form of *mental retardation* caused by a *chromo-*

somal abnormality; formerly called mongolism. Two types are recognized, based on the nature of the chromosomal aberration: the translocation type and the nondisjunction type. Physical findings include widely spaced eyes with slanting openings, small head with flattened occiput, lax joints, flabby hands, small ears, and *congenital* anomalies of the heart. See also *chromosome 21*.

DRG based payments See *diagnostic related groups*.

drive Basic urge, instinct, motivation; a term used to avoid confusion with the more purely biologic concept of *instinct*.

drug abuse See *drug dependence*.

drug dependence Habituation to, abuse of, and/or *addiction* to a chemical substance. Largely because of psychologic craving, the life of the drug-dependent person revolves around the need for the specific effect of one or more chemical agents on *mood* or state of consciousness. The term thus includes not only the addiction (which emphasizes the physiologic dependence), but also drug abuse (where the pathologic craving for drugs seems unrelated to physical dependence). Examples: alcohol, *opiates*, synthetic analgesics with morphinelike effects, *barbiturates*, other *hypnotics*, *sedatives* and some antianxiety agents, *cocaine*, psychostimulants, marijuana, and *psychotomimetic* drugs.

drug holiday Discontinuance of a therapeutic drug for a limited period of time. Sometimes used as a way of evaluating baseline behavior or as a means of controlling or reducing the dosage of psychoactive drugs and side effects.

drug-induced parkinsonism (pseudoparkinsonism) A reversible *syndrome* resembling the disease *parkinsonism*, resulting from the *dopamine*-blocking action of antipsychotic drugs. Pill-rolling movements are less common than in the naturally occurring disorder.

drug interaction The effects of two or more drugs taken simultaneously, producing an alteration in the usual effects of either drug taken alone. The interacting drugs may have a potentiating or additive effect and serious side effects may result. An example of drug interaction is alcohol and *sedative* drugs taken together, which may cause *central nervous system* depression.

drug levels See *blood levels*.

drug tolerance Repeated use of some substance or drug, often *narcotics*, so that larger and larger doses are required to produce the same physiologic and/or psychologic effect obtained previously by a smaller dose.

DSM See *Diagnostic and Statistical Manual of Mental Disorders*.

dummy British term for *placebo*.

Durham rule See *Table of Legal Terms*.

dyad A two-person relationship, such as the therapeutic relationship between doctor and patient in individual *psychotherapy*.

dynamic psychiatry The study of *psychiatry* from the point of view of motivation, emphasizing both psychologic meaning and biologic instincts as forces relevant to understanding human behavior in health, as well as illness. Contrast with *descriptive psychiatry*.

dynamics See *psychodynamics*.

dys- See *Table of Neurologic Deficits*.

dysarthria See *Table of Neurologic Deficits*.

dyscalculia See *learning disability*.

dysgraphia See *learning disability*.

dyskinesia Any disturbance of movement.

dyslexia Inability or difficulty in reading, including word-blindness and a tendency to reverse letters and words in reading and writing. See also *learning disability* and *alexia* in *Table of Neurologic Deficits*.

dysmnesia, dysmnesic syndrome General intellectual impairment secondary to defects of memory and orientation. See also *organic mental disorder*.

dyspareunia Painful sexual intercourse in the woman.

dysphagia Difficult or painful swallowing.

dysphonia Disorder of speech due to dysfunction of vocal cords.

dysphoria Unpleasant *mood*.

dyssocial behavior The behavior of persons who are not classifiable as antisocial personalities, but who are predatory and follow criminal pursuits. Formerly called sociopathic personalities. See also *personality disorders*.

dysthymic disorder See *depressive neurosis* under *neurosis*.

dystonia Acute tonic muscular spasms, often of the tongue, jaw, eyes, and neck, but sometimes of the whole body. Sometimes occurs during the first few days of antipsychotic drug administration.

E

eating disorder Marked disturbance in eating behavior. In *DSM-III-R*, eating disorders include *anorexia nervosa, bulimia, pica,* and *rumination* disorder of infancy.

echolalia See *Table of Neurologic Deficits*.

echopraxia Imitative repetition of the movements of another. Sometimes seen in *catatonic schizophrenia*.

ecology The study of the mutual relationship between people and their environment.

ecopsychiatry Scientific concept describing the basic and applied relationship between living things and their environment. These are assumed, by their presence or absence, to affect mental health.

ECT See *electroconvulsive treatment*.

ectomorphic See *constitutional types*.

educable Capable of achieving a fourth- or fifth-grade academic level; mildly mentally retarded (I.Q. 52 to 67)

EEG See *electroencephalogram*.

ego In *psychoanalytic* theory, one of the three major divisions in the model of the psychic apparatus, the others being the *id* and *superego*. The ego represents the sum of certain mental mechanisms, such as perception and memory, and specific *defense mechanisms*. It serves to mediate between the demands of primitive instinctual drives (the id), of internalized parental and social prohibitions (the superego), and of reality. The compromises between these forces achieved by the ego tend to resolve intrapsychic *conflict* and serve an adaptive and executive function. Psychiatric usage of the term should not be confused with common usage, which connotes self-love or selfishness.

ego alien See *ego-dystonic*.

ego analysis Intensive *psychoanalytic* study and analysis of the ways in which the *ego* resolves or attempts to deal with intrapsychic *conflicts*, especially in relation to the development of mental mechanisms and the maturation of capacity for rational thought and action. Modern *psychoanalysis* gives more emphasis to considerations of the defensive operations of the ego than did earlier techniques, which emphasized *instinctual* forces to a greater degree.

ego boundaries Refers to the ability of the intact ego to differentiate the real from the unreal.

egocentric Self-centered.

ego-dystonic Aspects of a person's behavior, thoughts, and attitudes viewed as repugnant or inconsistent with the total *personality*. Contrast with *ego-syntonic*.

ego ideal The part of the personality that comprises the aims and goals for the self; usually refers to the *conscious* or *unconscious* emulation of significant figures with whom one has identified. The ego ideal emphasizes what one should be or do in contrast to what one should not be or not do.

egomania See under *-mania*.

ego psychology The study and elucidation of those slowly changing functions known as psychic structures which usually shape, channel, and organize mental activity into meaningful and tolerable patterns of experience. The usual structures referred to in this sense are memory, speech, locomotion, cognition, drive, restraint, discharge, and the capacity to make judgments and decisions.

ego strength Ability to retain reality and manage the forces of the id and the superego.

ego-syntonic Aspects of a person's behavior, thoughts, and attitudes viewed as acceptable and consistent with the total *personality*. Contrast with *ego-dystonic*.

eidetic image Unusually vivid and apparently exact mental image; may be a memory, *fantasy*, or dream.

ejaculatory incompetence (impotence) Inability to reach orgasm and ejaculate during sexual intercourse despite adequacy of erection.

elaboration An *unconscious* process or expansion and embellishment of detail, especially with reference to a symbol or representation in a dream.

Electra complex An infrequently used term describing the pathologic relationship between a woman and a man based on unresolved developmental *conflicts* partially analogous to the *Oedipus complex* in a man.

electroconvulsive treatment (ECT) Use of electric current to induce convulsive seizures. Most effective in the treatment of *depression*. Introduced by Cerletti and Bini in 1938. Modifications are electronarcosis, which produces sleeplike states, and electrostimulation, which avoids convulsions. Used with anesthetics and muscle relaxants.

electroencephalogram (EEG) A graphic (voltage vs. time) depiction of the brain's electrical potentials recorded by scalp electrodes. It is used for diagnosis in neurologic and neuropsychiatric disorders and in neurophysiologic research. Sometimes used interchangeably with electrocorticogram and depth record, where the electrodes are in direct contact with brain tissue.

electromyogram (EMG) An electrophysiologic recording of muscle potentials that measures the amount and nature of muscle activity at the site from which the recording is taken.

electroshock treatment (EST) See *electroconvulsive treatment*.

electrostimulation See *electroconvulsive treatment*.

elopement A patient's unauthorized departure from a psychiatric facility.

EMG See *electromyogram*.

emotion A state of arousal determined by a set of subjective feelings, often accompanied by physiologic changes, which impels one toward action. Examples are fear, anger, love, hate, etc.

emotional disturbance See *mental disorder*.

emotional illness See *mental disorder*.

empathy Insightful awareness, including the meaning and significance of the feelings, *emotions*, and behavior of another person. Contrast with *sympathy*.

encephalitis Either acute or chronic inflammation of the brain caused by viruses, bacteria, spirochetes, fungi, and protozoa. Neurologic signs and *symptoms* and various mental and behavioral changes occur during the illness and may persist. See also *encephalopathy* and *organic mental disorder*.

encephalopathy Any of the metabolic, toxic, neoplastic, or degenerative diseases of the brain.

encopresis Incontinence of feces.

endemic See under *epidemiology*.

endocrine disorders Disturbances of the function of the ductless glands which may be metabolic in origin and may be associated with or aggravated by emotional factors, producing mental and behavioral disturbances in addition to physical signs.

endogenous depression See *depression*.

endomorphic See *constitutional types.*

endorphin A naturally produced chemical with morphine-like action; usually found in the brain and associated with the relief of pain. May be the body's own protection against pain.

engram A memory trace; a neurophysiologic process that accounts for persistence of memory.

enkephalin Endogenous opioid peptide found in the brain. See *endorphin.*

enuresis Nocturnal and daytime incontinence of urine.

enzyme An organic compound that interacts with a biologic substrate to form a new chemical, either commonly through the process of synthesis or through degradation. For example, the enzyme *monoamine oxidase* degrades *biogenic amines.*

epidemiology In *psychiatry,* the study of the incidence, distribution, prevalence, and control of *mental disorders* in a given population. Common terms in epidemiology are:

> **endemic** Native to or restricted to a particular area.

> **epidemic** The outbreak of a disorder that affects significant numbers of persons in a given population at any time.

> **pandemic** Occurring over a very wide area, in many countries, or universally. See also *incidence, point* and *period prevalence* in *Table of Research Terms.*

epilepsy A neurologic disorder characterized by periodic motor or sensory seizures or their equivalents, and sometimes accompanied by a loss of consciousness or by certain equivalent manifestations. May be idiopathic (no known organic cause) or symptomatic (due to organic lesions). Accompanied by abnormal electrical discharge which may be shown by *electroencephalogram*. See also *convulsive disorders*.

epileptic equivalent Episodic, sensory, or motor phenomena which a person with epilepsy may experience instead of convulsive seizures.

Jacksonian epilepsy Recurrent episodes of convulsive seizures or spasms without loss of consciousness localized in a part or region of the body; named after neurologist J. Hughlings Jackson (1835-1911).

major epilepsy (grand mal) Gross convulsive seizures with loss of consciousness and vegetative control.

minor epilepsy (petit mal) Nonconvulsive epileptic seizures or equivalents; may be limited only to momentary lapses of consciousness.

temporal lobe epilepsy An outdated term, now called complex partial seizures. It involves recurrent periodic disturbances of behavior, usually originating in the temporal lobes, during which the patient carries out movements that are often repetitive and highly organized but semiautomatic in character.

epinephrine One of the *catecholamines* secreted by the adrenal gland and by fibers of the *sympathetic nervous system*. It is responsible for many of the physical manifestations of *fear* and *anxiety*. Also known as adrenalin.

epistemology The theory of knowledge; the study of the method and grounds of knowledge.

Erikson, Erik H. (1902-   ) German-born lay *psychoanalyst* and child psychoanalyst noted for his work on *psychosocial development*; author of major studies of Luther and Ghandi.

erogenous zone An area of the body particularly susceptible to *erotic* arousal when stimulated, especially the oral, anal, and genital areas. Sometimes called erotogenic zone.

erotic *Consciously* or *unconsciously* invested with sexual feeling; sensually related.

erotomania See *-mania*.

erythrophobia See under *phobia*.

ESP See *extrasensory perception*.

ethnology A science that concerns itself with the division of mankind into races and their origin, distribution, relations, and characteristics.

ethology The scientific study of animal behavior; also the empirical study of human behavior.

etiology Causation, particularly with reference to disease.

euphoria An exaggerated feeling of physical and emotional well-being, usually of psychologic origin. Also seen in *organic mental disorders* and in toxic and drug-induced states. See also *bipolar disorder*.

event-related potential Electrical activity produced by the brain in response to a sensory stimulus or associated with the execution of a motor, cognitive, or psychophysiologic task. See also *evoked potential* and *electroencephalogram*.

evoked potential Electrical activity produced by the brain in response to any sensory stimulus; a more specific term than *event-related potential*. See also *electroencephalogram*.

executive ego function A *psychoanalytic* term for the ego's management of the mental mechanisms in order to meet the needs of the organism. See also *ego*.

exhibitionism Exposure of one's genitals to a person of the opposite sex in socially unacceptable situations. More common in males than in females. See also *paraphilia*.

existential psychiatry (existentialism) A school of *psychiatry* evolved from orthodox *psychoanalytic* thought; stresses the way in which a person experiences the phenomenologic world and takes responsibility for existence. Philosophically, it is *holistic* and self-deterministic in contrast to biologic or culturally deterministic points of view. See also *phenomenology* and *Table of Schools of Psychiatry*.

exogenous psychoses See *organic mental disorders*.

experiential group A group whose main purpose is concerned with sharing whatever happens in a spontaneous fashion.

expert witness See *Table of Legal Terms*.

explosive personality A disorder of impulse control in which several episodes of serious outbursts of relatively unprovoked aggression lead to assault on others or the destruction of property. There is no organic, epileptic, or any other *personality disorder* that might account for the behavior. Also called intermittent explosive personality.

extinction The weakening of a reinforced operant response as a result of ceasing *reinforcement*. See also *operant conditioning*. Also, the elimination of a conditioned response by repeated presentations of a conditioned stimulus without the unconditioned stimulus. See also *respondent conditioning*.

extrapyramidal syndrome A variety of signs and *symptoms*, including muscular rigidity, tremors, drooling, shuffling gait (parkinsonism); restlessness (*akathisia*); peculiar involuntary postures (*dystonia*); motor inertia (*akinesia*) and many other neurologic disturbances. Results from dysfunction of the *extrapyramidal system*. May occur as a reversible side effect of certain psychotropic drugs, particularly *phenothiazines*. See also *tardive dyskinesia* and *Table of Neurologic Deficits*.

extrapyramidal system The portion of the *central nervous system* responsible for coordinating and integrating various aspects of motor behavior or body movements.

extrasensory perception (ESP) Perception without recourse to the conventional use of any of the five physical senses. See also *telepathy*.

extroversion A state in which attention and energies are largely directed outward from the self as opposed to inward toward the self, as in *introversion*.

F

factitious disorders Disorders characterized by physical or psychologic *symptoms* that are intentionally produced or feigned. *See also Munchhausen syndrome.*

factor analysis A statistical technique that examines population clusters to extract patterns of commonality.

family therapy Treatment of more than one member of a family in the same session. The treatment may be supportive, directive, or interpretive. The assumption is that a *mental disorder* in one member of a family may be a manifestation of disorder in other members and may affect interrelationships and functioning.

fantasy An imagined sequence of events or mental images, e.g., daydreams, that serves to express *unconscious conflicts*, to gratify unconscious wishes, or to prepare for anticipated future events.

FDA *See Food and Drug Administration.*

fear Unpleasant emotional and physiologic response to recognized sources of danger, to be distinguished from *anxiety. See also phobia.*

feeblemindedness Obsolete term. *See mental retardation.*

femaleness Anatomic and physiologic features that relate to the female's procreative and nurturing capacities. *See also feminine.*

feminine A set of sex-specific social role behaviors unrelated to procreative and nurturing biologic functions. See also *gender identity*, *gender role*, and *femaleness*.

fetishism See *paraphilia*.

fixation The arrest of psychosocial development; may be considered pathologic, depending on the degree of intensity.

flagellation A *masochistic* or *sadistic* act in which one or both participants derive stimulation, usually *erotic*, from whipping or being whipped.

flexibilitas cerea See *cerea flexibilitas*.

flight of ideas Verbal skipping from one idea to another. The ideas appear to be continuous but are fragmentary and determined by chance or temporal associations. Sometimes seen in *bipolar disorder*.

flooding (implosion) A *behavior therapy* procedure for *phobias* and other problems involving maladaptive *anxiety*, in which anxiety producers are presented in intense forms, either in imagination or in real life. The presentations are continued until the stimuli no longer produce disabling anxiety.

folie à deux A condition in which two closely related persons, usually in the same family, share the same *delusions*. In *DSM-III-R* called induced psychotic disorder in recognition of the well known clinical fact that not all such instances involve shared delusions; they can also be manic, depressive, etc.

follow-up examination Repeated clinical assessment following discharge after inpatient or outpatient treatment.

Food and Drug Administration (FDA) One of a number of health administrations under the Assistant Secretary of Health of the U.S. Department of Health, Education and Welfare (in April 1980, Department of *Health and Human Services*) to set standards for, to license the sale of, and in general to safeguard the public from the use of dangerous drugs and food substances.

forensic psychiatry A branch of *psychiatry* dealing with legal issues related to mental disorders. See also *Table of Legal Terms*.

formal thought disorder See *thought disorder*.

formication The tactile *hallucination* or *illusion* that insects are crawling on the body or under the skin.

for-profit hospitals Hospitals owned and/or operated by physicians, other individuals, or a business corporation for the purpose of making a profit. Also called proprietary hospitals or investor-owned hospitals.

free association In *psychoanalytic* therapy, spontaneous, uncensored verbalization by the patient of whatever comes to mind.

free-floating anxiety Severe, generalized, persistent *anxiety* not specifically ascribed to a particular object or event and often a precursor of panic.

Freud, Anna (1895-1982) Austrian *psychoanalyst* and daughter of Sigmund *Freud*, noted for her contributions to the developmental theory of *psychoanalysis* and its applications to preventive work with children.

Freud, Sigmund (1856-1939) Founder of *psychoanalysis*. Most of the basic concepts of *dynamic psychiatry* are derived from his theories.

frigidity See *orgasmic dysfunction*.

fugue Personality *dissociation* characterized by *amnesia* and involving actual physical flight from the customary environment or field of *conflict*.

functional In medicine, changes in the way an organ system operates that are not attributed to known structural alterations. See also *functional disorder*.

functional disorder A disorder in which the performance or operation of an organ or organ system is abnormal, but not as a result of known changes in structure.

fusion In psychoanalysis, the joining together of instincts and objects.

G

GABA (gamma aminobutyric acid) The major *neurotransmitter* in the brain implicated in several psychiatric and neurologic conditions, most notably *Huntington's disease*. See also *disinhibition*.

galvanic skin response (GSR) The change in the electrical resistance of the skin in response to diverse stimuli; an easily measured variable widely used in experimental studies.

Ganser syndrome Sometimes called nonsense syndrome, syndrome of approximate answers, or prison psychosis (*e.g.*, two times two equal about five). Commonly used to characterize behavior of prisoners who seek, either *consciously* or *unconsciously*, to mislead others regarding their mental state in order to gain an advantage or escape responsibility.

gatekeeper A *primary care physician*, or occasionally another physician, to whom a defined insured population is assigned and who is required either to provide all health care or to authorize care from other specialists, if necessary, for the insured individual.

gateway drugs Term coined by Robert Dupont, M.D., to describe the three drugs that open up the gate to addiction: alcohol, cocaine, and marijuana.

Gault decision See *Table of Legal Terms*.

gender identity (core gender identity) The inner sense of *maleness* or *femaleness* which identifies the person as being male, female, or ambivalent. Differentiation of gender identity usually takes place in infancy and early childhood and is reinforced by the hormonal changes of puberty. Gender identity is distinguished from sexual identity, which is biologically determined. See also *gender role*; *transsexual*.

gender role The image a person presents to others and to the self that declares him or her to be boy or girl, man or woman. Gender role is the public declaration of *gender identity*, but the two do not necessarily coincide.

general paralysis (general paresis) A form of tertiary syphilis; an *organic mental disorder* occasionally associated with other neurologic signs of syphilitic involvement of the nervous system. Detectable with laboratory tests of the blood or spinal fluid. Sometimes known as GPI (general paralysis of the insane), an obsolete term.

generalized anxiety disorder A *DSM-III-R* term for anxiety *neurosis*. See also *neurosis*.

genes The fundamental units of heredity. Composed of DNA (deoxyribonucleic acid) and arranged in a characteristic linear sequence on *chromosomes* within cell nuclei. They determine the *genotype* of the individual.

genetic(s) In biology, pertaining to *genes* or to inherited characteristics. Also, in *psychiatry*, pertaining to the historical development of one's psychologic attributes or disorders.

genetic counseling Advice given to a prospective parental couple regarding the inheritance of a pathologic condition related to the couple's genetic endowment.

genetic endowment Inherited traits, potentials, and capacities.

genetic marker An observable trait or physical property that identifies or is associated with a specific region of the genetic material (DNA); a molecular signpost.

genital phase See *psychosexual development*.

genotype The total set of *genes* present at the time of conception, producing the genetic constitution. See also *phenotype*.

geriatric psychiatry A branch of *psychiatry* concerned with the psychologic aspects of the *aging* process and *mental disorders* of the aged.

geriatrics A branch of medicine dealing with the *aging* process and diseases of the aging human being.

gerontology The study of *aging*.

Gesell developmental schedules See *Table of Psychologic Tests*.

gestalt psychology A German school of *psychology* that emphasizes a total perceptual configuration and the interrelationships of its component parts. See also *Table of Schools of Psychiatry*.

Gilles de la Tourette syndrome A genetically determined *syndrome* usually beginning in early childhood characterized by repetitive *tics*, other movement disorders, uncontrolled grunts, unintelligible sounds, and occasionally verbal obscenities. Also known as Tourette's syndrome.

globus hystericus The disturbing sensation of a lump in the throat. See also *hysterical neurosis, conversion type*, under *neurosis*.

glossolalia Gibberish-like speech, or "speaking in tongues."

grand mal See *epilepsy*.

grandiosity Exaggerated belief or claims of one's importance or identity, often manifested by *delusions* of great wealth, power, or fame. See also *bipolar disorder* and *mania*.

grief Normal, appropriate emotional response to an external and *consciously* recognized loss; it is usually time-limited and subsides gradually. To be distinguished from *depression*.

group dynamics The interactions and interrelations among members of a therapy group and between members and the therapist. The effective use of group dynamics is essential in group treatment.

group practice A formal association of three or more physicians, or other health professionals, providing services. Income is pooled and redistributed to group members according to previous plans.

group psychotherapy Application of *psychotherapeutic* techniques to a group, including utilization of interactions of members of the group. Usually six to eight persons constitute a group and usually weekly sessions typically last 75 minutes or longer.

groups See *sensitivity group*; *group psychotherapy*.

guardianship See *Table of Legal Terms*.

guilt Emotion resulting from doing what one conceives of as wrong, thereby violating *superego* precepts; results in feelings of worthlessness and at times the need for punishment. See also *shame*,

H

habeas corpus See *Table of Legal Terms*.

halfway house A specialized residence for patients who do not require full hospitalization but who need an intermediate degree of care before returning to independent community living.

hallucination A sensory perception in the absence of an actual external stimulus. May occur in any of the senses.

hallucinogen A chemical agent that produces *hallucinations*. The term is used synonymously with *psychotomimetic*.

hallucinosis A condition in which the patient hallucinates in a state of clear consciousness. See also *alcoholic hallucinosis*.

haloperidol See *Table of Drugs Used in Psychiatry*.

Halstead-Reitan See *Table of Psychologic Tests*.

Health and Human Services A federal department established in 1953 as the Department of Health, Education, and Welfare to supervise and coordinate the following agencies: *Food and Drug Administration*, Office of Human Development, Public Health Service, Social Security Administration, *Alcohol, Drug Abuse and Mental Health Administration*, National Institutes of Health, Center for Disease Control, Health Care Financing Administration, Office of Children, Youth and Families, and Office of Smoking and Health. In 1979, a separate Department of Education was established and the remaining agencies became the Department of Health and Human Services.

health maintenance organization (HMO) A form of group practice by physicians and supporting personnel to provide comprehensive health services to an enrolled group of subscribers who pay a fixed premium to belong. Emphasis is on maintaining the health of the enrollees as well as treating their illnesses. HMO's must include psychiatric benefits to receive federal support.

hebephrenia See *schizophrenia, disorganized*.

hedonism Pleasure-seeking behavior. Contrast with *anhedonia*.

helplessness Inability to act on one's own behalf; inefficiency in making an impact on one's environment to create change.

heroin An illicit (in the United States) opioid commonly used by drug addicts. Heroin has a high physical dependence capacity; usually injected intravenously.

heterogeneity Dissimilarity in the genotypical structure of individuals originating through sexual reproduction.

HEW See *Health and Human Services*.

5HIAA (5-hydroxy-indoleacetic-acid) A major metabolite of *serotonin*, a *biogenic amine* found in the brain and other organs. Functional deficits of serotonin in the *central nervous system* have been implicated in certain types of major *mood disorders*.

histrionic See *personality disorders*.

holism An approach to the study of the individual in totality, rather than as an aggregate of separate physiologic, *psychologic*, and social characteristics.

homeostasis Self-regulating biologic and *psychologic* processes that maintain the equilibrium of the organism.

homosexual panic An acute and severe attack of *anxiety* based on *unconscious* conflicts involving *gender identity*.

homosexuality A preferential *erotic* attraction for members of the same sex.

homosexuality, ego-dystonic A sustained pattern of overt homosexual arousal which is a source of distress, since the person involved wishes to acquire or increase arousal patterns that allow heterosexual relations to be initiated or maintained. The term has been removed as a diagnostic entity in *DSM-III-R*.

homovanillic acid (HVA) A principal metabolite of *dopamine*, a *catecholamine* found in the brain and other organs.

hormone A discrete chemical substance secreted into the body fluids by an endocrine gland, which has a specific effect on the activities of other organs. See also *neurohormone*.

Horney, Karen (1883-1952) German *psychoanalyst* who emigrated to the United States in 1932, departed from orthodox *Freudian* thought and founded her own school, emphasizing cultural factors underlying the *neuroses*.

Hospital and Community Psychiatry An interdisciplinary monthly journal of the *American Psychiatric Association*.

hostility Actual or threatened aggressive contact, destructive in intent.

hotline Telephone assistance service for crisis intervention, usually focused on topics such as alcoholic binges, suicide, drugs, etc.

humiliation Sense of disgrace and shame often experienced in *depression*.

Huntington's disease (chorea) A hereditary and progressively degenerative disease of the *central nervous system* transmitted as an autosomal dominant trait. Onset is in adult life and is characterized by random movements (lurching, jerking) of the entire body. May include progressive mental deterioration and *psychosis*.

hyperactivity In *DSM-III-R*, called an *attention deficit disorder* (ADD); excessive motor activity, generally purposeful. It is frequently, but not necessarily, associated with internal tension or a neurologic disorder. Usually, the movements are more rapid than customary for the person.

hyperkinetic syndrome A disorder of childhood or *adolescence* characterized by overactivity, restlessness, distractibility, short attention span, and difficulties in learning and perceptual motor function. Believed in some cases to be associated with *minimal brain dysfunction*. In *DSM-III-R*, the official term is attention deficit-hyperactivity disorder and is classified as one of the disruptive behavior disorders.

hypersomnia Excessive amount of *sleep*, sometimes with confusion on waking.

hypertensive crisis Sometimes fatal effect of combining *monoamine oxidase inhibitors* with *tyramine* in food or with other sympathomimetic substances (e.g., cough remedies and nose drops).

hyperventilation Overbreathing sometimes associated with *anxiety* and marked by reduction of blood carbon dioxide, producing complaints of light-headedness, faintness, tingling of the extremities, palpitations, and respiratory distress.

hypesthesia Diminished sensitivity to tactile stimuli.

hypnagogic Referring to the semiconscious state immediately preceding sleep; may include *hallucinations*, which are of no pathologic significance.

hypnopompic Referring to the state immediately preceding awakening; may include *hallucinations*, which are of no pathologic significance.

hypnosis A phenomenon characterized by a person's ability to respond to appropriate suggestions by altering perception or memory; usually associated with the experience of behaving nonvolitionally. Factors determining the subject's responsivity include the nature of the preexisting relationship with the hypnotist, prior expectations, beliefs, and motivations concerning hypnosis and, most important, characterologic and individual differences.

hypnotic Any agent that induces *sleep*. Although *sedatives* and *narcotics* in sufficient dosage may produce sleep as an incidental effect, the term hypnotic is appropriately reserved for drugs employed primarily to produce sleep.

hypochondriasis A chronic maladaptive style of relating to the environment through preoccupation with shifting somatic concerns and *symptoms*, fear or conviction that one has a serious physical illness, seeking of medical treatment, inability to accept reassurance, and either hostile or dependent relationships with *caregivers* and family. In *DSM-III-R*, hypochondriasis is classified as a *somatization disorder*.

hypoglycemia Abnormally low level of blood sugar. See also *insulin coma treatment*.

hypomania A psychopathologic state and abnormality of *mood* falling somewhere between normal *euphoria* and *mania*. It is characterized by unrealistic optimism, pressure of speech and activity, and a decreased need for *sleep*. Some people show increased creativity during hypomanic states, while others show poor judgment, irritability, and irascibility. See also *bipolar disorder*.

hypothalamus The principal center in the forebrain for integration of visceral functions involving the *autonomic nervous system*.

hysterical personality See *histrionic* under *personality disorders*.

hysterics Lay term for uncontrollable emotional outbursts.

iatrogenic illness An illness unwittingly precipitated, aggravated, or induced by the physician's attitude, examination, comments, or treatment.

ICD-9 See *International Classification of Diseases*.

id In *Freudian* theory, the part of the personality that is the *unconscious* source of unstructured desires and drives. See also *ego, superego*.

idealization A mental mechanism, operating *consciously* or *unconsciously*, in which one overestimates an admired aspect or attribute of another.

ideas of reference Incorrect interpretation of casual incidents and external events as having direct reference to oneself. May reach sufficient intensity to constitute *delusions*.

idée fixe Fixed idea. Used in *psychiatry* to describe a *compulsive* drive, an *obsessive* idea, or a *delusion*.

identification A *defense mechanism*, operating unconsciously, by which a person patterns himself after some other person. Identification plays a major role in the development of one's personality and specifically of the *superego*. To be differentiated from imitation or role modeling, which is a *conscious* process.

identity A person's global role in life and the perception of his sense of self.

identity crisis A loss of the sense of the sameness and historical continuity of one's self and inability to accept or adopt the role one perceives as being expected by society; often expressed by isolation, withdrawal, extremism, rebelliousness, and negativity, and typically triggered by a combination of sudden increase in the strength of instinctual *drives* in a milieu of rapid social evolution and technologic change. See also *psychosocial development*.

idiopathic Of unknown cause.

idiot savant A person with gross mental retardation who nonetheless is capable of performing certain remarkable feats in sharply circumscribed intellectual areas, such as calendar calculation or puzzle-solving.

illusion A misperception of a real external stimulus. Example: the rustling of leaves is heard as the sound of voices. See also *hallucination*.

imago A term used by *Jung* for an *unconscious* mental image, usually idealized, of an important person in one's early history.

immediate memory The recall of perceived material within approximately five seconds after presentation.

implosion See *flooding*.

impotence The inability to achieve or maintain a penile erection of sufficient quality to engage in successful sexual intercourse. Two types are described by Masters and Johnson: in primary impotence, there has never been a successful sexual coupling; in secondary impotence, failure occurs following at least one successful union. Compare with *orgasmic dysfunction*.

imprinting A term in *ethology* referring to a process similar to rapid learning or behavioral patterning that occurs at critical points in very early stages of animal development. The extent to which imprinting occurs in human development has not been established.

impulse A psychic striving; usually refers to an *instinctual* urge.

impulse disorders A varied group of nonpsychotic disorders in which impulse control is weak. The impulsive behavior is usually pleasurable, irresistible, and *ego-syntonic*. Impulse disorders listed in *DSM-III-R* include pathological gambling, kleptomania, pyromania, intermittent explosive disorder, and trichotillomania.

inappropriate affect A display of emotion that is out of harmony with reality.

incest Sexual activity between close blood relatives, as father-daughter, mother-son, or between siblings.

incidence The frequency with which a disease occurs. See *Table of Research Terms*.

incompetency See *Table of Legal Terms*.

incorporation A primitive *defense mechanism*, operating *unconsciously*, in which the psychic representation of a person, or parts of the person, is figuratively ingested.

indigenous worker See *caregiver*.

individual psychology A system of psychiatric theory, research, and therapy developed by Alfred *Adler* which stresses *compensation* and *overcompensation* for inferiority feelings. See also *complex*.

individuation A process of differentiation, having for its goal the development of the individual personality.

indolamine One of a group of biogenic amines, e.g., serotonin, that contains an indole ring and amine group within its chemical structure.

indoles A group of *biogenic amines*.

industrial psychiatry *See occupational psychiatry.*

infant psychiatry An aspect of child psychiatry that deals with the diagnosis, treatment, and prevention of maladaptive psychologic functioning.

infantile autism *See autism.*

inferiority complex *See complex.*

informed consent Permission by the patient for a medical procedure based on understanding the nature of the procedure, the risks involved, the consequences of withholding permission, and alternative procedures. *See also Table of Legal Terms.*

infradian rhythms *See biologic rhythms.*

inhibition Behavioral evidence of an *unconscious* defense against forbidden *instinctual* drives; may interfere with or restrict specific activities.

insane Obsolete term for *mental disorder.*

insanity A vague term, now obsolete, for *psychosis.* Still used, however, in strictly legal contexts such as insanity defense. *See also Table of Legal Terms.*

insanity defense *See Table of Legal Terms.*

insecurity A feeling of helplessness against anxiety arising from uncertainty about one's goals, ideals, abilities, and relationships.

insight Self-understanding; the extent of a person's understanding of the origin, nature, and mechanisms of his maladaptive attitudes and behavior.

insomnia Inability to fall asleep, difficulty staying asleep, and/or early morning awakening.

instinct An inborn *drive*. The primary human instincts include self-preservation, sexuality, and—according to some proponents—*aggression*, the *ego instincts*, and hero or social instincts. *Freud* also postulated a *death instinct*.

institutionalization Admission of an individual to an institution, such as a nursing home, where he or she will reside for an extended period of time or indefinitely.

insulin coma treatment Injection of insulin in sufficient quantity to produce profound *hypoglycemia* (low blood sugar) resulting in *coma*. First used in 1933 in the treatment of *schizophrenia*; rarely used today.

intake The initial interview between a patient and a member of a psychiatric team in a mental health facility.

integration The useful organization and incorporation of both new and old data, experience, and emotional capacities into the *personality*. Also refers to the organization and amalgamation of functions at various levels of *psychosexual development*.

intellectualization The utilization of reasoning as a *defense* against confrontation with *unconscious* conflicts and their stressful *emotions*.

intelligence Capacity to learn and to utilize appropriately what one has learned. May be affected by *emotions*.

intelligence quotient (IQ) A numerical rating determined through psychologic testing that indicates the approximate relationship of a person's mental age (MA) to chronologic age (CA). Expressed mathematically as

$$IQ = \frac{MA}{CA} \times 100.$$ See also *Table of Psychologic Tests*.

International Classification of Diseases (ICD) The official list of disease categories issued by the World Health Organization; subscribed to by all member nations, who may assign their own terms to each ICD category. ICDA (International Classification of Diseases, adapted for use in the United States and prepared by the U.S. Public Health Service) represents the official list of diagnostic terms to be used for each ICD category in this country.

internship The first year of graduate medical education, which ordinarily is integrated into a full residency training program in a designated specialty.

interpersonal skills Effective adaptive behavior in relation to other persons.

interpretation The process by which the therapist brings the patient to an understanding of a particular aspect of his problems or behavior.

intoxication An organic mental disorder due to recent ingestion or presence in the body of a chemical agent, causing maladaptive behavior because of its effects on the *central nervous system*.

intrapsychic That which takes place within the *psyche* or mind.

intrapsychic conflict See *conflict.*

intravenous (IV) Within or into the veins.

introjection A *defense mechanism*, operating *unconsciously*, whereby loved or hated external objects are symbolically absorbed within oneself. The converse of *projection*. May serve as a defense against *conscious* recognition of intolerable hostile impulses. For example, in severe *depression*, the individual may unconsciously direct unacceptable hatred or *aggression* toward himself. Related to the more primitive *fantasy* of oral *incorporation.*

introspection Self-observation; examination of one's feelings, often as a result of psychotherapy.

introversion Preoccupation with oneself and accompanying reduction of interest in the outside world; the reverse of *extraversion.*

involutional melancholia A term formerly used to describe an agitated *depression* in a person of *climacteric* age. Currently, such patients are not distinguished from depressed patients of other age groups.

isolation A mechanism of defense operating *unconsciously* central to obsessive-compulsive phenomena in which the affect attached to an idea is rendered unconscious, leaving the conscious idea colorless and emotionally neutral.

isonome A signal or pathway in the brain that has similar effects on several different agencies.

J

Jacksonian epilepsy See *epilepsy*.

Janet, Pierre (1859-1947) French *psychiatrist* who formulated theories of hysterical conversion and dissociative conditions based on constitutional factors rather than psychodynamic ones. First to use the term *la belle indifférence*.

Joint Commission on Accreditation of Hospitals (JCAH) The agency that surveys and accredits hospitals and some other health facilities and programs as fulfilling their standards. See also *accreditation*.

Joint Commission on Mental Health of Children A multidisciplinary agency authorized by the U.S. Congress in 1965 (PL 89-97) and established in 1966 to study and report on the nation's "resources, methods, and practices for diagnosing or preventing emotional illness in children and of treating, caring for, and rehabilitating children with emotional illness." Its final report, "Crisis in Child Mental Health: Challenge for the 1970's," was published in 1969.

Joint Commission on Mental Illness and Health A multidisciplinary agency, incorporated in 1956 and representing 36 national agencies in the *mental health* and welfare fields. It conducted a five-year study of the mental health needs of the nation between 1956 and 1961 as authorized by the U.S. Congress in the Mental Health Study Act of 1955. The final report of the Joint Commission, "Action for Mental Health," led ultimately to legislation by Congress in 1963 authorizing and appropriating funds to facilitate the development of *com-*

munity mental health centers for the mentally ill and mentally retarded.

Jones, Ernest (1879-1958) English *psychoanalyst*, an early pupil of *Freud* and his principal biographer, who introduced *psychoanalysis* to the English-speaking world.

judgment Mental act of comparing choices between a given set of values in order to select a course of action.

Jung, Carl Gustav (1875-1961) Swiss *psychoanalyst*; founder of the school of *analytic psychology*. *See also anima, imago,* and *persona.*

K _____

kinesics The study of body posture, movement, and facial expressions.

Kirkbride, Thomas S. (1809-1883) American *psychiatrist*, one of the founders of the *American Psychiatric Association*. Noted for his pioneering contributions to mental hospital design.

Klein, Melanie (1882-1960) British pioneer in the *psychoanalysis* of children. Noted for her work on early childhood development, particularly infantile aggression and the origins of the *superego* in early infancy. *See also Table of Schools of Psychiatry.*

Kleine-Levin syndrome Periodic episodes of *hypersomnia*; first appears in *adolescence*, usually in boys, and is accompanied by *bulimia.*

kleptomania See *-mania.* Listed in *DSM-III-R* as an *impulse disorder.*

Klinefelter syndrome *Chromosomal* defect in males in which there is an extra X chromosome; manifestations may include underdeveloped testes, physical feminization, sterility, and mental retardation.

Klüver-Bucy syndrome A syndrome following bilateral temporal lobe removal consisting of loss of recognition of people, loss of fear, rage reactions, hypersexuality, excessive oral behavior, memory defect, and overreaction to visual stimuli.

koro See *culture-specific syndromes.*

Korsakoff syndrome See *alcoholic psychosis* and *Wernicke-Korsakoff syndrome.*

Kraepelin, Emil (1885-1926) German *psychiatrist* who developed an extensive systematic classification of mental illnesses. One of the first to delineate the concept of *dementia praecox* or *schizophrenia.* See also *descriptive psychiatry.*

Krafft-Ebing, Richard von (1840-1903) *Neuropsychiatrist* and student of sexual pathology, remembered for his now classic *Psychopathia Sexualis*, a pioneering study of sexual aberrations, published in 1886.

L

la belle indifférence Literally, "beautiful indifference." Seen in certain patients with *conversion* disorders who show an inappropriate lack of concern about their disabilities. See *hysterical neurosis, conversion type,* under *neurosis.* See also *Janet.*

labile Rapidly shifting *emotions;* unstable.

lapsus linguae A slip of the tongue due to *unconscious* factors.

latah See *culture-specific syndromes.*

latency period See *psychosexual development.*

latent content The hidden (*unconscious*) meaning of thoughts or actions, especially in dreams or fantasies. In dreams, it is expressed in distorted, disguised, condensed, and symbolic form.

learned helplessness A condition in which a person attempts to establish and maintain contact with another by adopting a helpless, powerless stance.

learning disability A *syndrome* affecting school age children of normal or above normal intelligence characterized by specific difficulties in learning to read (*dyslexia*), write (*dysgraphia*), and calculate (*dyscalculia*). The disorder is believed to be related to slow developmental progression of perceptual motor skills. See also *minimal brain dysfunction.*

lesbian *Homosexual* woman.

lethologica Temporary inability to remember a proper noun or name.

liaison nursing Consultation by clinical specialists in psychiatric nursing to nursing colleagues on issues of patient management in medical-surgical, parent-child, or geriatric settings.

liaison psychiatry See *consultation liaison psychiatry*.

libido The psychic *drive* or energy usually associated with the sexual *instinct*. (Sexual is used here in the broad sense to include pleasure and love-object seeking.)

limbic system An area in the brain associated with the control of emotion, eating, drinking, and sexual activity.

lithium carbonate An alkali metal, the salt of which is used in the treatment of acute *mania* and as a maintenance medication to help reduce the duration, intensity, and frequency of recurrent affective episodes, especially in *bipolar disorders*.

living will A document devised as a means by which terminally ill people can set limits on the effort to keep them alive beyond the point they would themselves choose.

lobotomy A type of *psychosurgery* in which one or more nerve tracts on the cerebrum are severed. This procedure is now rarely used in the U.S.A.

locus coeruleus A small area in the brainstem that is considered to be a key brain center for anxiety and fear.

logorrhea Uncontrollable, excessive talking.

long-term memory The recall of events or information from the distant past. Contrast with *immediate memory*.

loosening of associations A disturbance of thinking in which ideas shift from one subject to another in an oblique or unrelated manner. The speaker is unaware of the disturbance. When loosening of associations is severe, speech may be incoherent. Contrast with *flight of ideas*.

LSD (lysergic acid diethylamide) A potent *hallucinogen* that produces psychotic *symptoms* and behavior. Symptoms may include *hallucinations, illusions*, body and time-space distortions, and, less commonly, intense panic or mystical experiences.

lumbar puncture The insertion of a needle between two of the lumbar vertebrae into the meningeal sac around the base of the spinal cord to obtain cerebrospinal fluid for diagnostic purposes.

Luria, Alexander Romanovich (1902-1977) Russian neuropsychologist who developed a treatment for aphasia, combining physical and psychologic techniques for victims of brain trauma.

magical thinking A conviction that thinking equates with doing. Occurs in dreams in children, in primitive peoples, and in patients under a variety of conditions. Characterized by lack of realistic relationship between cause and effect.

magnetic resonance imaging (MRI) A technique for imaging anatomical structures which involves placing subjects in a strong magnetic field and then, by use of magnetic gradients and brief radio frequency pulses, determining the resonance characteristics at each point in the area to be studied. Used to detect structural or anatomical abnormalities, such as brain tumor and incipient multiple sclerosis. See also *brain imaging*.

maintenance drug therapy Reducing the dosage of a therapeutic drug after it has reached its maximum efficacy and sustaining it at the minimum level to prevent a relapse.

major affective disorders In *DSM-III* a group of disorders in which there is a prominent and persistent disturbance of *mood* (*depression* or *mania*) and a full *syndrome* of associated symptoms. The category includes bipolar disorder and major depression. The disorders are usually episodic but could be chronic. In *DSM-III-R* the term major affective disorders has been changed to mood disorders and is divided into *bipolar* and *depressive disorders*.

major epilepsy (grand mal) See under *epilepsy*.

maladjustment Unsuccessful attempts at *adaptation*.

maleness Anatomic and physiologic features that relate to the male's procreative capacity. See also *masculine*.

malingering Deliberate simulation or exaggeration of an illness or disability in order to avoid an unpleasant situation or to obtain some type of personal gain. See also *factitious disorder, compensation neurosis,* and *secondary gain.*

mania A *mood* disorder characterized by excessive elation, hyperactivity, *agitation,* and accelerated thinking and speaking. Sometimes manifested as *flight of ideas.* Mania is seen in *mood disorders* and in certain *organic mental disorders.*

-mania Formerly used as a nonspecific term for any kind of "madness." Currently used as a suffix to indicate a morbid preoccupation with some kind of idea or activity, and/or a *compulsive* need to behave in some deviant way. Some examples are:

egomania Pathologic preoccupation with self.

erotomania Pathologic preoccupation with *erotic* fantasies or activities.

kleptomania Compulsion to steal.

megalomania Pathologic preoccupation with *delusions* of power or wealth.

monomania Pathologic preoccupation with one subject.

necromania Pathologic preoccupation with dead bodies.

nymphomania Abnormal and excessive need or desire in the woman for sexual intercourse; see also *satyriasis.*

pyromania Morbid compulsion to set fires; an *impulse disorder*.

trichotillomania Compulsion to pull out one's hair; an *impulse disorder*.

maniac Imprecise, sensational, and misleading term for an emotionally disturbed person. Usually implies violent behavior. Not specifically referable to any psychiatric diagnostic category.

manic depressive illness A term often used synonymously with *bipolar disorder*, as defined in *DSM-III-R*.

manifest content The remembered content of a dream or fantasy, as contrasted with *latent content*, which is concealed and distorted.

manipulation A behavior pattern characterized by attempts to exploit interpersonal contact.

MAOI See *monamine oxidase inhibitor*.

marijuana Dried leaves and flowers of *Cannabis sativa* which induces somatic and psychic changes when smoked or ingested in sufficient quantity.

marital therapy A treatment whose goal is to ameliorate problems of married couples. Various psychodynamic, sexual, ethical, and economic aspects of marriage are considered. Husband and wife are usually seen individually or conjointly. A broader term is couples therapy, which encompasses unmarried couples.

masculine A set of sex-specific social role behaviors that are unrelated to procreative biologic function. See also *gender identity*, *gender role*, and *maleness*.

masculine protest Term coined by *Adler* to describe a striving to escape identification with the feminine role. Applies primarily to women but may also be noted in men.

masochism Pleasure derived from physical or psychologic pain inflicted either by oneself or by others. When it is *consciously* sought as a part of the sexual act or as a prerequisite to sexual gratification, it is classified as a *paraphilia*. It is the converse of *sadism*, although the two tend to coexist in the same person.

maternal deprivation The result of the premature loss or absence of the mother, or the lack of proper mothering.

maturational crises Predictable life events or turning points that occur for most individuals.

mean See *Table of Research Terms*.

median See *Table of Research Terms*.

Medicaid A program of medical services, financed jointly by the state and federal governments, designed for those who cannot afford regular medical services. For programs receiving federal support, the services paid include: inpatient and outpatient hospital services; other laboratory and x-ray services; skilled nursing facility and home health services for those over 21; early and periodic screening, diagnosis, and treatment for those under 21; family planning; and physician services.

medical audit See *audit*.

medical ethics The moral code adopted by health professionals in assigning primary value to their patient's needs and interests.

medical record A written document which contains sufficient information to identify the patient clearly and to justify the diagnosis and treatment and to document the results accurately.

medical review Review by a team composed of physicians and other appropriate health personnel of the conditions and need for care, including a medical evaluation.

Medicare The hospital insurance system and the supplementary medical insurance for the aged and certain categories of disabled created by the 1965 amendments to the Social Security Act. The insurance, Parts A and B, provides the same hospital benefits in general hospitals for psychiatric conditions as for other conditions but limits benefits in psychiatric hospitals to 190 days during a lifetime.

megalomania See *-mania*.

megavitamin therapy See *orthomolecular treatment*.

melancholia A term used since antiquity to refer to a severe form of *depression*. In *DSM-III-R*, the term major depression with melancholia refers to a severe depression that includes loss of pleasure, *mood* worse in the morning, *psychomotor retardation* or *agitation*, weight loss, and *insomnia*. See *major affective disorders*.

memory The ability, process, or act of remembering or recalling, especially the ability to reproduce what has been learned or explained.

menarche The onset of menstruation.

mendacity Pathologic lying.

mental age (MA) A measure of mental ability as determined by psychologic tests.

mental deficiency See *mental retardation*.

mental disease See *mental disorder*.

mental disorder An illness with psychologic or behavioral manifestations and/or impairment in functioning due to a social, psychologic, genetic, physical/chemical, or biologic disturbance. The disorder is not limited to relations between the person and society. The illness is characterized by *symptoms* and/or impairment in functioning.

mental health A state of being, relative rather than absolute. The best indices of mental health are simultaneous success at working, loving, and creating with the capacity for mature and flexible resolution of conflicts between *instincts*, *conscience*, important other people, and reality.

mental illness See *mental disorder*.

mental retardation Significantly subaverage general intellectual functioning existing concurrently with deficits in adaptive behavior and manifested during the developmental period.

mental status The level and style of functioning of the *psyche*, including a person's intellectual functioning and emotional, attitudinal, psychologic, and personality aspects. The term is commonly used to refer to the results of the examination of the patient's mental state.

mental status examination The process of estimating psychologic and behavioral function by observing the patient, eliciting his description of self, and formally questioning him. Included in the examination are (1) evaluation and assessment of any psychiatric condition present, including provisional diagnosis and prognosis, determination of degree of impairment, suitability for treatment, and indications for particular types of therapeutic intervention; (2) formulation of the personality structure of the subject, which may suggest the historical and developmental antecedents of whatever psychiatric condition exists; (3) estimation of the ability and willingness to participate appropriately in treatment. The mental status is reported in a series of narrative statements describing such things as *affect*, speech, thought content, perception, and *cognitive* functions. The mental status examination is part of the general examination of all patients, although it may be markedly abbreviated in the absence of *psychopathology*.

mescaline An alkaloid originally derived from the peyote cactus, resembling *amphetamine* and adrenalin chemically; used to induce altered perceptions. Also used by Indians of the Southwest in religious rites. See *Table of Commonly Abused Drugs*.

mesmerism Early term for hypnosis. Named after Anton Mesmer (1733-1815).

mesomorphic See *constitutional types*.

metapsychiatry The interface between *psychiatry* and such psychic phenomena as *parapsychology*, mysticism, altered states of consciousness, and nonmedical healing.

metapsychology The branch of theoretical or speculative *psychology* that deals with the significance of mental processes; the nature of the mind-body relationship; the origin, purpose, and structure of the mind; and similar hypotheses that are beyond the realm of empirical verification.

methadone A synthetic *narcotic*. It may be used as a substitute for heroin, producing a less socially disabling *addiction* or aiding in the withdrawal from heroin. It may be abused. See also *narcotic blocking drugs* and *Table of Commonly Abused Drugs.*

Metrazol shock treatment A rarely used treatment in which a convulsive seizure is produced by intravenous injection of Metrazol (known as Cardiazol in Europe). Introduced by von Meduna in 1934.

Meyer, Adolf (1866-1950) American *psychiatrist*, professor of psychiatry at Johns Hopkins University; introduced the concept of *psychobiology*. See *Table of Schools of Psychiatry.*

MHPG (3-methoxy-4-hydroxphenylglycol) A major metabolite of brain *norepinephrine* excreted in urine.

middle age Conventionally considered to occur between 40 and 60 years of age and primarily defined by *psychosocial* rather than by physiologic events.

mid-life crisis The set of problems that arise when individuals discover visible signs that they are aging and become preoccupied with the realization.

migraine A *syndrome* characterized by recurrent, severe, and usually one-sided headaches; often associated with nausea, vomiting, and visual disturbances.

milieu therapy Socioenvironmental therapy in which the attitudes and behavior of the staff of a treatment service and the activities prescribed for the patients are determined by the patients' emotional and interpersonal needs. This therapy is an essential part of all inpatient treatment.

minimal brain dysfunction (MBD) A disturbance of children, adolescents, and perhaps adults, without signs of major neurologic or psychiatric disturbance. Characterized by decreased attention span, distractibility, increased activity, impulsivity, emotional *lability*, poor motor integration, disturbances in perception and disorders of language development. See also *learning disability*.

Minnesota Multiphasic Personality Inventory (MMPI) See *Table of Psychologic Tests*.

minor epilepsy (petit mal) See under *epilepsy*.

Mitchell, S. Weir (1830-1914) American *neurologist* who described *causalgia* and developed a once popular "rest cure" for emotional disorders.

M'Naghten rule See *Table of Legal Terms*.

mode See *Table of Research Terms*.

molecular biology An aspect of biology that seeks to understand, explain, or rationalize biologic phenomena in terms of molecular (or chemical) interactions.

molecular psychiatry A science that deals specifically with brain chemicals that are released in minute quantities by one neuron to mediate its communication with other neurons. See also *neuroscience*.

molecular psychology See *molecular psychiatry*.

molecule A very small mass of matter; a chemical combination of two or more atoms which form a specific chemical substance.

mongolism See *Down's syndrome*.

monoamine An amine containing only one amino group.

monoamine oxidase (MAO) An enzyme that breaks down biogenic amines (neurotransmitters), rendering them inactive. Found in many body organs, including the brain. Inhibition of this enzyme by certain antidepressant drugs (MAOI's) may result in alleviation of depressed states. See also *biogenic amines* and *Table of Drugs Used in Psychiatry*.

monoamine oxidase inhibitor (MAOI) A group of antidepressant drugs that inhibit the enzyme *monoamine oxidase* in the brain and raise the levels of *biogenic amines*. See *Table of Drugs Used in Psychiatry*.

monomania See *-mania*.

monozygotic twins Twins who develop from a single fertilized ovum; identical twins.

mood A pervasive and sustained emotion that, in the extreme, markedly colors one's perception of the world.

Common examples of mood include *depression*, elation, and anger. See also *affect*.

mood disorders A DSM-III-R term for *major affective disorders*.

mood swing Fluctuation of a person's emotional tone between periods of elation and periods of depression.

moral treatment A philosophy and technique of treating mental patients that prevailed in the first half of the nineteenth century and emphasized removal of restraints, humane and kindly care, attention to religion, and performance of useful tasks in the hospital.

mourning Reaction to a loss of a love object (important person, object, role, status, or anything considered part of one's life) consisting of a process of emotional detachment from that object which frees the subject to find other interests and enjoyments.

MRI See *magnetic resonance imaging*.

multiple personality A term used by *Morton Prince* for a rare type of dissociative reaction in which the person adopts two or more personalities. In *DSM-III-R*, classified as a *dissociative disorder*. See also *hysterical neurosis, dissociative type*, under *neurosis*.

Münchhausen syndrome (pathomimicry) A rare, difficult to treat disorder. Sufferers habitually attempt to hospitalize themselves with self-defined or self-induced pathology, yearning for a surgical remedy. No definitive *etiology* has been established. In *DSM-III-R*, this syndrome is diagnosed as chronic *factitious disorder* with physical symptoms.

mutation A change in hereditary constitution that causes genetically transmissible permanent differences. May occur spontaneously or may be induced by such agents as high-energy radiation. See also *genes*.

mutism Refusal to speak for *conscious* or *unconscious* reasons.

mysophobia See *phobia*.

N _____

naloxone A pure, potent, but short-acting narcotic *antagonist* with no *agonistic* effects of its own; the drug of choice in the treatment of narcotic overdose. Its short duration of action (2-4 hours) makes it generally inappropriate for chronic treatment of narcotic *addiction*, but large doses have been used to produce narcotic blockade for up to 18 hours in addicts involved in day-treatment programs. See also *narcotic blocking drugs*.

narcissism (narcism) Self-love as opposed to object-love (love of another person). In *psychoanalytic* theory, *cathexis* (investment) of the psychic representation of the self with *libido* (sexual interest and energy). An excess interferes with relations with others. To be distinguished from egotism, which carries the connotation of self-centeredness, selfishness, and conceit. Egotism is but one expression of narcissism.

narcoanalysis See *narcosynthesis*.

narcolepsy Uncontrollable, recurrent, brief episodes of *sleep* associated with excessive daytime sleepiness, *cataplexy*, sleep paralysis, *hypnagogic hallucinations*, and often disturbed nocturnal sleep.

narcosis Stupor of varying depth induced by certain drugs.

narcosynthesis Psychotherapeutic treatment under partial *anesthesia*, such as induced by *barbiturates*. Originally used to treat acute mental disorders occurring in a military combat setting.

narcotic Any opiate derivative drug, natural or synthetic, that relieves pain or alters *mood*. May cause *addiction*. See also *drug dependence*, *hypnotic*, *sedative*.

narcotic blocking drugs (narcotic antagonists). Agents structurally similar to the opiates and probably occupying the same receptor sites in the *central nervous system*. In sufficient doses they block the effects of opiate drugs by competing for their receptor sites. If given after opiate dependence has developed, they will precipitate an acute *abstinence* syndrome.

National Alliance for the Mentally Ill (NAMI) An organization whose membership consists of parents and relatives of mentally ill patients and former patients whose main objective is for better and more sustained care. Its trustees and chapter officers engage in active lobbying and in education projects.

National Institute of Mental Health (NIMH) An institute within ADAMHA responsible for programs dealing with mental health.

National Mental Health Association (NMHA) Leading voluntary citizens' organization in the mental health field; formerly called the National Association for Mental Health; founded in 1909 by *Clifford W. Beers* as the National Committee for Mental Hygiene.

necromania See under *-mania*.

negativism Opposition or resistance, either covert or overt, to outside suggestions or advice. May be seen in *schizophrenia*.

neologism In *psychiatry*, a new word or condensed combination of several words coined by a person to express a highly complex idea not readily understood by others; seen in *schizophrenia* and *organic mental disorders*.

nervous breakdown A nonmedical, nonspecific euphemism for a *mental disorder*.

neurochemistry The branch of chemistry that deals with the alterations that occur within the nervous system.

neuroendocrinology The science of the relationships between the nervous system (particularly the brain) and the endocrine system. Of particular importance is the action of the hypothalamus, which stimulates or inhibits the pituitary secretion of hormones.

neurohormone A chemical messenger usually produced within the *hypothalamus*, carried to the pituitary, and then to other cells within the *central nervous system (CNA)*. Neurohormones are similar to *neurotransmitters* except that they interact with a variety of cells, whereas neurotransmitters interact only with other neurons.

neuroleptic An antipsychotic drug. See also *Table of Drugs Used in Psychiatry*.

neuroleptic malignant syndrome A rare, idiosyncratic, and sometimes fatal reaction to high-potency neuroleptic drugs; most likely a result of dopamine blockade on the basal ganglia and hypothalamus. Symptoms include muscle rigidity and high fever.

neurologic disorders See *Table of Neurologic Deficits*.

neurologist A physician with postgraduate training and experience in the field of organic diseases of the nervous system whose professional work focuses primarily on this area. Neurologists also receive training in *psychiatry*.

neurology The branch of medical science devoted to the study, diagnosis, and treatment of organic diseases of the nervous system.

neuron A nerve cell.

neurophysiology The study of the function of the nervous system.

neuropsychiatry The medical specialty that combines neurology and psychiatry, emphasizing the somatic substructure on which emotions are based and the organic disturbances of the *central nervous system* that give rise to mental disorders.

neuroreceptors Binding sites in the *central nervous system* for psychoactive drugs.

neuroscience The study of normal brain function and the neural substrates of behavior, especially mental disorders and maladaptive behavior. Neuroscience is an interdisciplinary field that includes investigation in areas such as physiology, anatomy, *psychology*, *biochemistry*, *psychiatry*, and computer science.

neurosis In common usage, emotional disturbances of all kinds other than *psychosis*. It implies subjective psychologic pain or discomfort beyond what is appropriate in the conditions of one's life. The meaning of the term has been changed since it was first introduced into standard nomenclature. In *DSM-III-R*, the term signifies a limited number of specific diagnostic categories, all of which are attributed to maladaptive ways of dealing with *anxiety* or internal *conflict*. As currently used, some clinicians limit the term to its descriptive meaning, *neurotic disorder*, whereas others include the concept of a specific *etiologic* process. Common neuroses and their *DSM-III-R* equivalents are:

anxiety neurosis Chronic and persistent apprehension manifested by autonomic hyperactivity (sweating, palpitations, dizziness, etc.), musculoskeletal tension, and irritability. Somatic symptoms may be prominent. Referred to in *DSM-III-R* as either generalized anxiety disorder or panic disorder. See also *anxiety*.

depersonalization neurosis Feelings of unreality and of estrangement from the self, body, or surroundings. Different from the process of *depersonalization*, which may be a manifestation of anxiety or of another mental disorder. Referred to as depersonalization disorder in *DSM-III-R*.

depressive neurosis Excessive reaction of *depression* due to an internal *conflict* or to an identifiable event such as loss of a loved person or a cherished possession. In *DSM-III-R*, referred to as dysthymic disorder.

hysterical neurosis, conversion type Disorders of the special senses or the voluntary nervous system, such as blindness, deafness, *anesthesia*, *paresthesia*, pain, paralysis, and impaired muscle coordination. A patient with this disorder may show *la belle indifférence* to the symptoms, which may actually provide *secondary gains* by winning sympathy or relief from unpleasant responsibilities. Referred to in *DSM-III-R* as conversion disorder or psychogenic pain disorder. *See also conversion*.

hysterical neurosis, dissociative type Alterations in the state of consciousness or in identity, producing such *symptoms* as *amnesia*.

obsessive compulsive neurosis Persistent intrusion of unwanted and uncontrollable *ego-dystonic* thoughts, urges, or actions. The thoughts may consist of single words, ruminations, or trains of thought that are seen as nonsensical. The actions may vary from simple movements to complex rituals, such as repeated handwashing. *See also compulsion*. Referred to as obsessive compulsive disorder in *DSM-III-R*.

phobic neurosis An intense fear of an object or situation that the person consciously recognizes as harmless. Apprehension may be experienced as faintness, fatigue, palpitations, perspiration, nausea, tremor, and even *panic*. *See also phobia, social phobia*. In *DSM-III-R*, phobias are classified as agoraphobia without panic, simple phobia, or social phobia. Social phobia is the fear of situations such as public speaking or eating in public; simple phobias are fears of specific things such as animals, insects, or darkness.

neurotic disorder A *mental disorder* in which the predominant disturbance is a distressing *symptom* or group of symptoms which one considers unacceptable and alien to one's personality. There is no marked loss of *reality testing*; behavior does not actively violate gross social norms although it may be quite disabling. The disturbance is relatively enduring or recurrent without treatment and is not limited to a mild transitory reaction to *stress*. There is no demonstrable organic *etiology*. In *DSM-III-R*, the neurotic disorders are included in *affective, anxiety, somatoform, dissociative,* and *psychosexual* disorders. See also *neurotic process*.

neurotic process A specific *etiologic* process involving the following sequence: *unconscious conflicts* between opposing wishes or between wishes and prohibitions lead to *unconscious* perception of anticipated danger or *dysphoria*, which leads to use of *defense mechanisms* that result in either *symptoms*, *personality* disturbance, or both. See also *neurotic disorder* and *neurosis*.

neurotoxin A substance that is poisonous or destructive to nerve tissue.

neurotransmitter A chemical found in the nervous system (e.g. *dopamine*, noradrenaline, and *serotonin*) that facilitates the transmission of impulses across *synapses* between *neurons*. Disorders in the brain physiology of neurotransmitters have been implicated in the pathogenesis of several psychiatric illnesses, particularly *major affective disorders* and *schizophrenia*.

night hospital See *partial hospitalization*.

night terror (pavor nocturnus) See *sleep terror disorder*.

nightmare (dream anxiety attack) *Anxiety*-provoking dream occurring during *REM sleep*. Contrast with *sleep terror disorder*.

nihilistic delusion The *delusion* of nonexistence of the self, part of the self, or of some object in external reality.

norepinephrine A *catecholamine neurotransmitter* related to *epinephrine*. It is found in both the peripheral and *central nervous systems*. Functional excesses in the brain have been implicated in the pathogenesis of *manic* states; deficits, in certain depressive states. Also called noradrenaline. See also *biogenic amines*.

nosology Science of the classification of disorders, usually medical.

not-for-profit hospital A hospital which exists for the purpose of public service, rather than for the profit of its owners. Such a hospital may be partly or wholly publicly owned. Also called a voluntary hospital.

NREM sleep See *sleep*.

nuclear family Immediate members of a family.

nuclear magnetic resonance (NMR) See *magnetic resonance imaging* (MRI); also *brain imaging*.

null hypothesis See *Table of Research Terms*.

nursing-care plan A means of providing nursing personnel with information about the needs and therapeutic strategy for each patient.

nymphomania See under *-mania*.

O

object relations The emotional bonds between one person and another, as contrasted with interest in and love for the self; usually described in terms of capacity for loving and reacting appropriately to others.

obsession A persistent, unwanted idea or impulse that cannot be expunged by logic or reasoning.

obsessive compulsive neurosis See under *neurosis*.

occupational psychiatry (industrial psychiatry) A field of *psychiatry* concerned with the diagnosis and prevention of *mental illness* in industry, with the return of the psychiatric patient to work, and with psychiatric aspects of absenteeism, *accident proneness*, *alcoholism* and *substance abuse*, retirement, and related phenomena. Often works in consultation to an employees assistance program (EAP).

occupational therapy An adjunctive therapy that utilizes purposeful activities as a means of altering the course of illness. The patient's relationship to staff and to other patients in the occupational therapy setting is often more therapeutic than the activity itself.

Oedipus complex Attachment of the child to the parent of the opposite sex, accompanied by envious and *aggressive* feelings toward the parent of the same sex. These feelings are largely *repressed* (i.e., made *unconscious*) because of the fear of displeasure or punishment by the parent of the same sex. In its original use, the term applied only to the boy or man.

onanism Coitus interruptus. The term is sometimes used interchangeably with masturbation.

ontogenetic Pertaining to the development of the individual. Contrast with *phylogenetic*.

operant conditioning (instrumental conditioning) A process by which the results of the person's behavior determine whether the behavior is more or less likely to occur in the future. See also *respondent conditioning* and *shaping*.

opiate Any chemical derived from opium; relieves pain and produces a sense of well-being.

oral phase See *psychosexual development*.

organic brain syndrome See *organic mental disorder*.

organic disease A disease characterized by demonstrable structural or biochemical abnormality in an organ or tissue. Sometimes imprecisely used as an antonym for *functional disorder*.

organic mental disorder Transient or permanent dysfunction of the brain, caused by a disturbance of physiologic functioning of brain tissue at any level of organization—structural, hormonal, biochemical, electrical, etc. *DSM-III-R* recognizes the following organic brain syndromes: *delirium*, *dementia*, amnestic syndrome, organic anxiety syndrome, organic delusional syndrome, organic hallucinosis, organic mood syndrome, organic personality syndrome, and mixed or atypical brain syndrome, all of which are classified according to *etiology* or pathophysiology. Causes are associated with aging, toxic substances, or a variety of physical disorders.

orgasm Sexual climax; peak psychophysiologic response to sexual stimulation.

orgasmic dysfunction Inability of the woman to achieve *orgasm* through physical stimulation. Masters and Johnson describe two types. In primary orgasmic dysfunction, the woman has never had an orgasm through any physical contact, including masturbation. In situational orgasmic dysfunction, there has been at least one instance of orgasm through physical contact. Compare with *impotence*. In *DSM-III-R*, orgasmic dysfunction is not limited to females.

orientation Awareness of one's self in relation to time, place, and person.

Original Thirteen The thirteen founding fathers of the Association of Medical Superintendents of American Institutions for the Insane, 1844-1891, and The American Medico-Psychological Association, 1892-1919. See also *American Psychiatric Association*.

orphan drugs Drugs that the pharmaceutical companies do not wish to develop either because they cannot be patented (e.g., lithium), because they are used only in rare conditions by very few people, or for a variety of legitimate economic reasons. In such cases, the federal government will work with the companies to make the drugs available to those who need them.

orthomolecular treatment (megavitamin therapy) An approach based on the assumption that "for every twisted mind there is a twisted molecule" and that in some way psychiatric illness, and perhaps other illnesses, are due to biochemical abnormalities, resulting in increased needs for specific substances, such as vitamins. This treatment is of unknown and unproved efficacy.

orthopsychiatry An approach that involves the collaborative effort of *psychiatry, psychology, psychiatric social work*, and other behavioral, medical, and social sciences in the study and treatment of human behavior in the clinical setting. Emphasis is placed on preventive techniques to promote healthy emotional growth and development, particularly of children.

outpatient A patient who is receiving ambulatory care at a hospital or other health facility without being admitted to the facility.

overcompensation A *conscious* or *unconscious* process in which a real or imagined physical or psychologic deficit generates exaggerated correction. Concept introduced by *Adler.*

overdetermination The concept of multiple *unconscious* causes of an *emotional* reaction or *symptom*.

P _____

pandemic See under *epidemiology*.

panic Sudden, overwhelming *anxiety* of such intensity that it produces terror and physiologic changes.

panic disorder Discrete periods of intense fear or discomfort. Listed in *DSM-III-R* as an *anxiety* disorder, with or without agoraphobia.

panphobia Fear of everything. See *phobia*.

paranoia A rare condition characterized by the gradual development of an intricate, complex, and elaborate system of thinking based on (and often proceeding logically from) misinterpretation of an actual event. A person with paranoia often considers himself endowed with unique and superior ability. Despite its chronic course, this condition does not seem to interfere with thinking and personality. To be distinguished from *schizophrenia, paranoid type*.

paranoid A lay term commonly used to describe an overly suspicious person. The technical use of the term refers to people with *paranoid ideation* or to a type of *schizophrenia* or a class of disorders. See also *delusional (paranoid) disorders*.

paranoid disorders See *delusional (paranoid) disorders*.

paranoid ideation Suspiciousness or nondelusional belief that one is being harassed, persecuted, or unfairly treated.

paraphilia A condition in which persistent and repetitive sexually arousing *fantasies* of an unusual nature are associated with either preference for or use of a nonhuman object for sexual arousal, repetitive sexual activity with human beings involving real or simulated suffering or humiliation, or repetitive sexual activity with nonconsenting partners.

parapraxis A faulty act, blunder, or lapse of memory such as a slip of the tongue or misplacement of an article. According to *Freud*, these acts are caused by *unconscious* motives.

paraprofessional A trained aide who assists a professional person, usually in a medical setting.

parapsychology The study of sensory and motor phenomena shown by some human beings (and some animals) that occur without the mediation of the known sensory and motor organs. The data of parapsychology are not accounted for by the tenets of conventional science.

parasympathetic nervous system The part of the *autonomic nervous system* that controls the life-sustaining organs of the body under normal, danger-free conditions. See also *sympathetic nervous system*.

parataxic distortion *Sullivan's* term for inaccuracies in judgment and perception, particularly in interpersonal relations, based on the observer's need to perceive subjects and relationships in accordance with a pattern set by earlier experience. Parataxic distortions develop as a *defense* against *anxiety*.

paresis Weakness of organic origin; incomplete paralysis; term often used instead of *general paralysis*.

paresthesia Abnormal tactile sensation, often described as burning, pricking, tickling, tingling, or creeping.

parkinsonism A neurologic disorder characterized by rapid, coarse tremor, pill-rolling movements, masklike facies, cogwheel rigidity, drooling, *akinesia*, bradykinesia, or gait disturbances. Associated with *do-*

pamine depletion in the basal ganglia. See also *drug-induced parkinsonism*.

partial hospitalization A psychiatric treatment program for patients who require hospitalization only during the day, overnight, or on weekends.

passive-aggressive personality See *personality disorders*.

passive-dependent personality See *dependent* personality under *personality disorders*.

pastoral counseling The use of psychologic principles by clergymen trained to assist members of their congregation who seek help with emotional problems.

pathognomonic A *symptom* or group of symptoms that are specifically diagnostic or typical of a disease.

Pavlov, Ivan Petrovich (1849-1936) Russian neurophysiologist noted for his research on conditioning. Awarded Nobel Prize in Medicine (1904) for his work on the physiology of digestion.

pavor nocturnus See *sleep terror disorder*.

pederasty *Homosexual* anal intercourse between men and boys with the latter as the passive partners. The term is used less precisely to denote male homosexual anal intercourse.

pedophilia A *paraphilia* involving sexual activity of adults with children as the objects. It may involve any form of heterosexual or *homosexual* intercourse.

peer review Review by panels of physicians, and sometimes allied health professionals, of services rendered by other physicians. See also *professional standards review organization* and *utilization review committee*.

peer review organization (PRO) A system that determines the appropriateness and reasonableness of medical care under the Medicare program.

pellagra A vitamin B3 (nicotinamide) deficiency that may be a cause of major mental *symptoms* such as *delusions* and impaired thinking, as well as physical symptoms such as dermatitis.

penis envy In *psychoanalytic* theory, envy by the female child of the male child's genitals.

perception Mental processes by which intellectual, sensory, and emotional data are organized logically or meaningfully.

perseveration See *Table of Neurologic Deficits*.

persona A Jungian term for the personality mask or facade that each person presents to the outside world, as distinguished from the person's inner being or *anima*. See *Jung*.

personality The characteristic way in which a person thinks, feels, and behaves; the ingrained pattern of behavior that each person evolves, both *consciously* and *unconsciously*, as the style of life or way of being in adapting to the environment.

personality disorders Deeply ingrained, inflexible, maladaptive patterns of relating, perceiving, and thinking of sufficient severity to cause other impairment in functioning or distress. Personality disorders are generally recognizable by *adolescence* or earlier, continue throughout adulthood, and become less obvious in middle or old age. Some personality disorders cited in *DSM-III-R* are:

antisocial A lack of socialization along with behavior patterns that bring a person repeatedly into conflict with society; incapacity for significant loyalty to others or to social values; callousness; irresponsibility; impulsiveness; and inability to feel guilt or learn from experience or punishment. Frustration tolerance is low and such people tend to blame others or give plausible rationalizations for their behavior. Characteristic behavior appears before age 15, although the diagnosis may not be apparent until adulthood.

borderline A disorder that includes, in interpersonal relationships, inappropriate, intense, uncontrolled anger; identity disturbance; instability of *affect*; intolerance of being alone; physically self-damaging acts; and feelings of emptiness.

compulsive Restricted ability to express warm and tender emotions; preoccupation with rules, order, organization, efficiency, and detail; excessive devotion to work and productivity to the exclusion of pleasure; indecisiveness.

dependent Inducing others to assume responsibility for major areas of one's life; subordinating one's own needs to those of others on whom one is dependent to avoid any possibility of independence; lack of self confidence.

histrionic Excitability, emotional instability, over-reactivity, and attention-seeking and often seductive self-dramatization, whether or not the person is aware of its purpose. People with this disorder are immature, self-centered, vain, and unusually dependent. Sometimes referred to as hysterical personality.

narcissistic Grandiose sense of self-importance or uniqueness; preoccupation with fantasies of limitless success; need for constant attention and admiration; and disturbances in interpersonal relationships such as lack of *empathy*, exploitativeness, and relationships that vacillate between the extremes of overidealization and devaluation.

paranoid Pervasive and long-standing suspiciousness and mistrust of others; hypersensitivity and scanning of the environment for clues that selectively validate prejudices, attitudes, or biases. Stable psychotic features such as *delusions* and *hallucinations* are absent.

passive-aggressive Aggressive behavior manifested in passive ways such as obstructionism, pouting, procrastination, intentional inefficiency, and obstinacy. The *aggression* often arises from resentment at failing to find gratification in a relationship with an individual or institution upon which the individual is overdependent.

schizoid Manifested by shyness, oversensitivity, social withdrawal, frequent daydreaming, avoidance of close or competitive relationships and eccentricity. Persons with this disorder often react to disturbing experiences with apparent detachment and are unable to express hostility and ordinary aggressive feelings.

schizotypal The essential features are various oddities of thinking, perception, communication, and behavior not severe enough to meet the criteria for *schizophrenia*. No single feature is invariably present. The distur-

bance in thinking may be expressed as *magical thinking,
ideas of reference,* or *paranoid ideation.* Perceptual
disturbances may include recurrent *illusions,* depersonalization, or derealization. Often there are marked
peculiarities in communication; concepts may be expressed unclearly or oddly, using words deviantly, but
never to the point of *loosening of associations* or inco-
herence. Frequently, but not invariably, the behavioral
manifestations include social isolation and constricted
or inappropriate *affect* that interferes with rapport in
face-to-face interaction.

persuasion A therapeutic approach based on direct suggestion and guidance intended to influence favorably
patients' attitudes, behaviors, and goals.

perversion An imprecise term used to designate sexual
variance. See also *paraphilia.*

petit mal See *epilepsy.*

phallic phase See *psychosexual development.*

phantom limb A phenomenon frequently experienced
by amputees in which sensations, often painful, appear
to originate in the amputated extremity.

pharmacokinetics The study of the process and rates
of drug distribution, metabolism, and disposition in the
organism.

phencyclidine (PCP) See *Table of Commonly Abused
Drugs.*

phenomenology The study of occurrences or happen-
ings in their own right, rather than from the point of
view of inferred causes; specifically, the theory that be-

havior is determined, not by external reality as it can be described objectively in physical terms, but rather by the way in which the subject perceives that reality at any moment. See also *existential psychiatry*.

phenothiazine derivatives A group of *psychotropic* drugs that, chemically, have in common a phenothiazine configuration but differ from one another through variations in other components of the molecule. As a group of drugs, the phenothiazines are also known as antipsychotic drugs or *neuroleptics*. See *Table of Drugs Used in Psychiatry*.

phenotype The observable attributes of an individual; the physical manifestations of the *genotype*.

phenylketonuria (PKU) A genetic, metabolic disturbance characterized by an inability to convert phenylalanine to tyrosine. Results in the abnormal accumulation of chemicals that interfere with brain development. Treatable by diet when detected in early infancy. If untreated, mental retardation results. Also known as phenylpyruvic oligophrenia.

phobia An *obsessive*, persistent, unrealistic, intense *fear* of an object or situation. The fear is believed to arise through a process of displacing an internal (*unconscious*) conflict to an external object symbolically related to the conflict. See also *displacement*. Some of the common phobias are (add "abnormal fear of" to each entry):

achluophobia Darkness

acrophobia Heights

agoraphobia Open spaces or leaving the familiar setting of the home

ailurophobia Cats

algophobia Pain

androphobia Men

autophobia Being alone or solitude

bathophobia Depths

claustrophobia Closed spaces

cynophobia Dogs

demophobia Crowds

erythrophobia Blushing; sometimes used to refer to the blushing itself

gynophobia Women

hypnophobia Sleep

mysophobia Dirt and germs

panphobia Everything

pedophobia Children

xenophobia Strangers

phrenology Theory of the relationship between the structure of the skull and mental traits.

phylogenetic Pertaining to the development of the species. Contrast with *ontogenetic*.

pia mater A delicate fibrous membrane closely enveloping the brain and spinal cord.

Piaget, Jean (1896-1980) Swiss *psychologist* noted for his theoretical concepts of and research on the mental development of children. See also *cognitive development*.

piblokto See *culture-specific syndromes*.

pica An eating disorder consisting of the craving and eating of unusual foods or other substances. Seen in a variety of medical conditions, pregnancy, and emotional disturbances.

Pick's disease A presenile degenerative disease of the brain, possibly hereditary, affecting the cerebral cortex focally, particularly the frontal lobes. *Symptoms* include intellectual deterioration, emotional instability, and loss of social adjustment. See also *Alzheimer's disease*.

Pinel, Phillipe (1746-1826) French physician-reformer who pioneered in abolishing the use of restraints for the mentally ill.

piperazine See *Table of Drugs Used in Psychiatry*.

piperidine See *Table of Drugs Used in Psychiatry*.

placebo A material without pharmacologic activity but identical in appearance to an active drug. Used in pharmacologic research as a method of determining the actual effects of the drug being tested. See also *Table of Research Terms*.

placebo effect The production or enhancement of psychologic or physical effects using pharmacologically inactive substances administered under circumstances in which suggestion leads the subject to believe a particular effect will occur. See also *Table of Research Terms*.

plaques Certain areas of the brain that have undergone a specific form of degeneration. Senile plaques (neuritic plaques) consist of a central amyloid core surrounded by a less densely staining zone consisting of abnormal neurons, with many axonal and dendritic processes and masses of paired helical filaments. In Alzheimer's disease, they are particularly dense in the amygdaloid complex and the hippocampus. The relation between the abnormal protein fibers inside neurons (the paired helical filaments) and those outside the cells (i.e., amyloid) is currently unknown. The AD-DP gene, which codes for the beta-amyloid protein that accumulates in the blood vessel walls and in the neuronal tissue in both Alzheimer's and aged Down's brains, maps to *chromosome 21*.

plasma level See *blood levels*.

play therapy A treatment technique utilizing the child's play as a medium for expression and communication between patient and therapist.

pleasure principle The *psychoanalytic* concept that people instinctually seek to avoid pain and discomfort and strive for gratification and pleasure. In personality development theory, the pleasure principle antedates and subsequently comes in conflict with the *reality principle*.

polyphagia Pathologic overeating. Also known as *bulimia*.

polysomnography The all-night recording of a variety of physiologic parameters (e.g., brain waves, eye movements, muscle tonus, respiration, heart rate, penile tumescence) in order to diagnose *sleep*-related disorders.

porphyria A metabolic disorder characterized by the excretion of porphyrins in the urine and accompanied by attacks of abdominal pain, peripheral neuropathy, and a variety of mental symptoms. Some types are precipitated by *barbiturates* and alcohol.

positron emission tomography (PET scanning) A *brain-imaging* technique that permits one to evaluate regional metabolic differences by looking at radio-isotope distribution. By using positron-emitting isotopes of glucose, oxygen, neurotransmitters, or drugs, one can localize sites of increased (or decreased) metabolic turnover, receptor findings, or blood flow in a wide variety of neurologic or psychiatric conditions. The visual display is similar to *computerized axial tomography* (CAT scanning).

postpartum psychosis An inexact term for any *psychosis* (organic or functional) occurring within 90 days after childbirth.

posttraumatic stress disorder Disorder developing after experiencing a psychologically distressing event. It is characterized by reexperiencing the event and by overresponsiveness to, or involvement with, stimuli that recall the event. Also called "Vietnam vet's disease." Depression, startle reactions, flashback phenomena, and dissociative episodes are present.

potency The male's ability to carry out sexual relations. Often used to refer specifically to the capacity to have and maintain adequate erection of the penis during sexual intercourse. See also *impotence*.

preconscious Thoughts that are not in immediate awareness but that can be recalled by *conscious* effort.

pregenital In *psychoanalysis*, refers to the period of early childhood before the genitals have begun to exert the predominant influence in the organization or patterning of sexual behavior. Oral and anal influences predominate during this period. See also *psychosexual development*.

premature ejaculation Undesired ejaculation occurring immediately before or very early in sexual intercourse. The rapidity of ejaculation may prevent the woman from achieving sexual satisfaction or reaching orgasm.

presenile dementia In *DSM-III-R* called primary degenerative dementia, presenile onset. See also *Alzheimer's disease, Pick's disease*.

pressured speech Rapid, accelerated, frenzied speech. Sometimes it exceeds the ability of the vocal musculature to articulate, leading to jumbled and cluttered speech; at other times it exceeds the ability of the listener to comprehend as the speech expresses a *flight of ideas* (as in *mania*) or an unintelligible jargon.

prevalence Frequency of a disorder, used particularly in *epidemiology* to denote the total number of cases for a unit of population at a given time.

prevention (preventive psychiatry) In traditional medical usage, the prevention or prophylaxis of a disorder. In *community psychiatry*, the meaning of prevention encompasses the amelioration, control, and limitation of disease. Prevention is often categorized as follows:

primary prevention Measures to prevent a *mental disorder* (e.g., by nutrition, substitute parents, etc.).

secondary prevention Measures to limit a disease process (e.g., through early case-finding and treatment).

tertiary prevention Measures to reduce impairment or disability following a disorder (e.g., through *rehabilitation* programs).

primal scene In *psychoanalytic* theory, the real or fancied observation by the infant of parental or other heterosexual intercourse.

primary care physician Usually a general practitioner or specialist in family practice, internal medicine, pediatrics, or occasionally, obstetrics and gynecology, who serves as an initial contact for patients in managed health systems.

primary diagnosis The condition established after study to be the most severe condition for which the patient receives treatment.

primary gain The relief from emotional *conflict* and the freedom from *anxiety* achieved by a *defense mechanism*. Contrast with *secondary gain*.

primary process In *psychoanalytic* theory, the generally unorganized mental activity characteristic of the *unconscious*. It is marked by the free discharge of energy and excitation without regard to the demands of environment, reality, or logic. See also *secondary process.*

Prince, Morton (1845-1929) American *psychiatrist* and *neurologist* known for his work on *multiple personalities.*

principal diagnosis The condition established after study to be chiefly responsible for the admission of the patient to the hospital or for outpatient treatment.

prison psychosis See *Ganser syndrome.*

privileged communication See *Table of Legal Terms.*

problem-oriented record A simple conceptual framework to expedite and improve medical records. It contains four logically sequenced sections: the data base, the problem list, plans, and follow-up.

problem-solving A specific form of intellectual activity used when an individual faces a situation he is unable to handle in terms of past learning. Problem-solving strategies are considered crucial in any psychotherapeutic endeavor.

process schizophrenia See under *schizophrenia.*

prodrome (precursor) An early or premonitory symptom of a disease or a disorder.

professional standards review organization (PSRO) A physician sponsored organization charged with comprehensive and ongoing review of services provided under Medicare, Medicaid, and maternal and child health programs. The object of this review is to determine for purposes of reimbursement under these programs, whether services are medically necessary; provided in accordance with professional criteria, norms, and standards; and in the case of institutional services, rendered in appropriate settings. See also *peer review organization* (PRO).

prognosis The prediction of the future course of an illness.

projection A *defense mechanism*, operating *unconsciously*, in which what is emotionally unacceptable in the self is unconsciously rejected and attributed (projected) to others.

projective tests Psychologic diagnostic tests in which the test material is unstructured so that any response will reflect a *projection* of some aspect of the subject's underlying *personality* and *psychopathology*. See also *Table of Psychologic Tests*.

prolactin A hormone secreted by the pituitary that promotes lactation in the female and may stimulate testosterone secretion in the male. Prolactin secretion is in part controlled by inhibiting and releasing factors in the brain. Because *dopamine* is involved in the brain's inhibition of prolactin secretion, the measurement of serum prolactin has been proposed as a way of judging the efficacy of specific antipsychotic drugs that have been thought to act primarily by blocking dopamine's effects.

pseudodementia A *syndrome* in which *dementia* is mimicked or caricatured by functional psychiatric illness. *Symptoms* and responses to *mental status examination* questions are similar to those found in verified cases of dementia. In pseudodementia, the chief diagnosis to be considered in the differential is *depression* in an older person vs. cognitive deterioration on the basis of organic brain disease.

psyche The mind.

psychedelic A term applied to any of several drugs that may induce *hallucinations* and psychotic states, including the production of distortions of time, sound, color, etc. Among the more commonly used psychedelics are *LSD*, marijuana, mescaline, psilocybin. See also *Table of Commonly Abused Drugs*.

psychiatric illness See *mental disorder*.

Psychiatric News The biweekly newspaper of the *American Psychiatric Association*.

psychiatric nurse Any nurse employed in a psychiatric hospital or other psychiatric setting who has special training and experience in the management of psychiatric patients. Sometimes the term is used to denote only those nurses who have a master's degree in psychiatric nursing.

psychiatric social worker See *social worker, psychiatric*.

psychiatrist A licensed physician who specializes in the diagnosis, treatment, and prevention of mental and emotional disorders. Training encompasses a medical degree and four years or more of approved postgraduate training. For those who wish to enter a subspecialty such as child psychiatry, *psychoanalysis*, administration, and the like, additional training is essential.

psychiatry The medical science that deals with the origin, diagnosis, prevention, and treatment of *mental disorders*.

psychic determinism See *determinism*.

psychoactive substance use disorder See *drug dependence*.

psychoanalysis A theory of the *psychology* of human development and behavior, a method of research, and a system of *psychotherapy*, originally developed by *Freud*. Through analysis of *free associations* and *interpretation* of dreams, *emotions* and behavior are traced to the influence of repressed instinctual *drives* and defenses against them in the *unconscious*. Psychoanalytic treatment seeks to eliminate or diminish the undesirable effects of unconscious *conflicts* by making the *analysand* aware of their existence, origin, and inappropriate expression in current emotions and behavior. See also *Table of Schools of Psychiatry*.

psychoanalyst A person, usually a *psychiatrist*, who has had training in *psychoanalysis* and who employs the techniques of psychoanalytic theory.

psychobiology A school of psychiatric thought which views biologic, psychologic, and social life experiences of a person as an integrated unit. Associated with *Adolf Meyer*, who introduced the term in the United States in 1915. See also *Table of Schools of Psychiatry*.

psychodrama A technique of group *psychotherapy* conceived and practiced by the late J.L. Moreno, M.D., in which individuals express their own or assigned emotional problems in dramatization.

psychodynamics The systematized knowledge and theory of human behavior and its motivation, the study of which depends largely upon the functional significance of *emotion*. Psychodynamics recognizes the role of *unconscious* motivation in human behavior. The science of psychodynamics assumes that one's behavior is determined by past experience, genetic endowment, and current reality.

psychoendocrinology The study of the psychological effects of neuroendocrinologic activity. For example, it is known that the release and inhibition of pituitary hormones are mediated in part by brain monoamines, disorders of which have been implicated in the pathogenesis of various psychiatric illnesses.

psychogenesis Production or causation of a *symptom* or illness by mental or psychic factors as opposed to organic ones.

psychogenic pain disorder In *DSM-III-R* called *somatoform disorder*; pain in which adequate physical findings are absent and in which there is evidence that psychologic factors play a causal role. See *somatoform disorder*.

psychohistory An approach to history that examines events within a psychologic framework.

psychoimmunology The study of the connection between the brain and emotions and the immune system.

psycholinguistics The study of factors affecting activities involved in communicating and comprehending verbal information. See also *kinesics*.

psychologic autopsy Post-mortem evaluations of the psychodynamics leading to a person's suicide.

psychologic tests See *Table of Psychologic Tests.*

psychologist A person who holds a degree in *psychology* from an accredited program. Providers of psychologic services are licensed under applicable state law, whereas those who teach or do research are usually exempt from licensure requirements.

psychology An academic discipline, a profession, and a science dealing with the study of mental processes and behavior of people and animals.

psychology, analytic See *analytic psychology* and *Jung.*

psychology, individual See *individual psychology* and *Adler.*

psychometry The science of testing and measuring mental and psychologic ability, efficiency potentials, and functioning, including *psychopathologic* components. See also *Table of Psychologic Tests.*

psychomotor Combined physical and mental activity.

psychomotor agitation Generalized physical and emotional overactivity in response to internal and/or external stimuli, as in *hypomania.*

psychomotor retardation A generalized slowing of physical and emotional reactions. Specifically, the slowing of movements such as eye-blinking; frequently seen in depression.

psychoneurosis See *neurosis.*

psychopathic personality An early term for antisocial personality. Such persons are sometimes referred to as psychopaths. See also *personality disorders.*

psychopathology The study of the significant causes and processes in the development of *mental disorders.* Also the manifestations of mental disorders.

psychopharmacology The study of the effects of psychoactive drugs on behavior in both animals and people. Clinical psychopharmacology more specifically includes both the study of drug effects in patients and the expert use of drugs in the treatment of psychiatric conditions.

psychophysiologic disorders A group of disorders characterized by physical *symptoms* that are affected by emotional factors and involve a single organ system, usually under *autonomic nervous system* control. Symptoms are caused by physiologic changes that normally accompany certain emotional states, but the changes are more intense and sustained. Frequently called *psychosomatic* disorders. These disorders are usually named and classified according to the organ system involved (e.g., gastrointestinal, respiratory). In *DSM-III-R*, such cases would be diagnosed as psychologic factors affecting physical condition. The specific physical condition is diagnosed and recorded separately.

psychosexual development A series of stages from infancy to adulthood, relatively fixed in time, determined by the interaction between a person's biologic *drives* and the environment. With resolution of this interaction, a balanced, reality-oriented development takes place; with disturbance, *fixation* and *conflict* ensue. This disturbance may remain latent or give rise to characterologic or behavioral disorders. The stages of development are:

oral The earliest of the stages of infantile psychosexual development, lasting from birth to 12 months or longer. Usually subdivided into two stages: the oral *erotic*, relating to the pleasurable experience of sucking, and the oral sadistic, associated with aggressive biting. Both oral eroticism and *sadism* continue into adult life in disguised and sublimated forms, such as the character traits of demandingness or pessimism. Oral conflict, as a general and pervasive influence, might underlie the psychologic determinants of addictive disorders, *depression*, and some functional psychotic disorders.

anal The period of *pregenital* psychosexual development, usually from one to three years, in which the child has particular interest and concern with the process of defecation and the sensations connected with the anus. The pleasurable part of the experience is termed anal eroticism. See also *anal character*.

phallic The period from about 2 1/2 to 6 years, during which sexual interest, curiosity, and pleasurable experience center about the penis in boys, and in girls, to a lesser extent, the clitoris.

oedipal Overlapping some with the phallic stage, this phase (ages four to six) represents a time of inevitable conflict between the child and parents. The child must desexualize the relationship to both parents in order to retain affectionate kinship with both of them. The process is accomplished by the internalization of the images of both parents, thereby giving more definite shape to the child's *superego*. With this internalization largely completed, the regulation of self-esteem and moral behavior comes from within.

psychosexual dysfunction A disorder characterized by an inhibition in sexual desire; sexual excitement, *orgasm, premature ejaculation, dyspareunia,* or *vaginismus* may also be present. In *DSM-III-R*, called *sexual disorders* to reflect more accurately the fact that a biogenic component is often present.

psychosis A major *mental disorder* of *organic* or *emotional* origin in which a person's ability to think, respond emotionally, remember, communicate, interpret reality, and behave appropriately is sufficiently impaired so as to interfere grossly with the capacity to meet the ordinary demands of life. Often characterized by *regressive* behavior, inappropriate *mood*, diminished impulse control, and such abnormal mental content as *delusions* and *hallucinations*. The term is applicable to conditions having a wide range of severity and duration. See also *schizophrenia, bipolar disorder, depression, organic mental disorder*, and *reality testing*.

psychosocial development Progressive interaction between a person and his environment through stages beginning in infancy, as primarily described by *Erikson*. Specific developmental tasks involving social relations and the role of social reality are faced by a person at phase-specific developmental points. The early tasks parallel stages of *psychosexual development*; the later tasks extend through adulthood. Successful and unsuccessful solutions to each task are listed below with the corresponding chronologic period and psychosexual stage where applicable. See also *cognitive development*.

Task Solutions	Chronologic Period	Psychosexual Stage
trust vs. mistrust	infancy	oral
autonomy vs. shame, doubt	early childhood (toddler)	anal
initiative vs. guilt	preschool	phallic (Oedipal)
industry vs. inferiority	school age	latency
identity vs. identity diffusion	adolescence	
intimacy vs. isolation	young adulthood	genital
generativity vs. self-absorption	adulthood	
integrity vs. despair	mature age	

psychosomatic The constant and inseparable interaction of the *psyche* (mind) and the *soma* (body). Most commonly used to refer to illnesses in which the manifestations are primarily physical with at least a partial emotional etiology. See also *psychophysiologic disorders*.

psychosurgery Surgical intervention to sever fibers connecting one part of the brain with another or to remove or to destroy brain tissue with the intent of modifying or altering severe disturbances of behavior, thought content, or *mood*. Such surgery may also be undertaken for the relief of intractable pain.

psychotherapist A person trained to treat mental, emotional, or behavioral disorders.

psychotherapy A process in which a person who wishes to relieve *symptoms* or resolve problems in living or is seeking personal growth enters into an implicit or explicit contract to interact in a prescribed way with a psychotherapist. See also *brief psychotherapy*.

psychotic depression See *depression*.

psychotomimetic Literally, mimicking a *psychosis*. Used to refer to certain drugs such as *LSD* or *mescaline*, which may produce psychotic states.

psychotropic A term used to describe drugs that have a special action upon the *psyche*. See also *Table of Drugs Used in Psychiatry*.

pyromania See under *-mania*.

q-sort See *Table of Research Terms*.

quality assurance Activities and programs intended to assure the quality of care in a defined medical setting or program. Such programs must include educational components intended to remedy identified deficiencies in quality.

R

random A statistical term that denotes accuracy by chance or without attention to selection or planning. See also *Table of Research Terms*.

Rank, Otto (1884-1939) Viennese lay *psychoanalyst* and early follower of *Freud*. "The Trauma of Birth," his major book, was published in 1924. He emigrated to the United States in 1935 and strongly influenced the Philadelphia Child Guidance Center and the University of Pennsylvania School of Social Work.

rape Sexual assault; forced sexual intercourse without the partner's consent.

rapport The feeling of harmonious accord and mutual responsiveness that contributes to the patient's confidence in the therapist and willingness to work cooperatively. To be distinguished from *transference*, which is *unconscious*.

rationalization A *defense mechanism*, operating *unconsciously*, in which an individual attempts to justify or make *consciously* tolerable by plausible means, feelings, behavior, or motives that otherwise would be intolerable. Not to be confused with conscious evasion or dissimulation. See also *projection*.

Ray, Isaac (1807-1881) A founder of the *American Psychiatric Association* whose "Treatise on the Medical Jurisprudence of Insanity" was the pioneer American work in *forensic psychiatry*.

reaction formation A *defense mechanism*, operating *unconsciously*, in which a person adopts *affects*, ideas, attitudes, and behaviors that are the opposites of impulses he harbors either *consciously* or unconsciously (e.g., excessive moral zeal may be a reaction to strong but *repressed* asocial impulses).

reactive depression See *depression*.

reactive schizophrenia See *schizophrenia*.

reality principle In *psychoanalytic* theory, the concept that the *pleasure principle*, which represents the claims of *instinctual* wishes, is normally modified by the demands and requirements of the external world. In fact, the reality principle may still work on behalf of the pleasure principle, but it reflects compromises and allows for the postponement of gratification to a more appropriate time. The reality principle usually becomes more prominent in the course of development but may be weak in certain psychiatric illnesses and undergo strengthening during treatment.

reality testing The ability to evaluate the external world objectively and to differentiate adequately between it and the internal world. Falsification of reality, as with massive *denial* or *projection*, indicates a severe disturbance of *ego* functioning and/or the perceptual and memory processes upon which it is partly based. See also *psychosis*.

recall The process of bringing a memory into *consciousness*. Recall is often used to refer to the recollection of facts, events, and feelings that occurred in the immediate past.

receptor A specialized area on a nerve membrane, a blood vessel, or a muscle that receives the chemical stimulation that activates or inhibits the nerve, blood vessel, or muscle.

reciprocal inhibition In *behavior therapy*, the hypothesis that if *anxiety*-provoking stimuli occur simultaneously with the inhibition of anxiety (e.g., relaxation), the bond between those stimuli and the anxiety will be weakened.

reference, delusion of (idea of) See *ideas of reference*.

regional cerebral blood flow (RCBF) A measurement obtained by using a noninvasive technique such as radioactive xenon to chart brain blood flow. See also *brain imaging*.

regression Partial or symbolic return to more infantile patterns of reacting or thinking. Manifested in a wide variety of circumstances such as normal *sleep*, play, physical illness, and in many *mental disorders*.

rehabilitation In psychiatry, the methods and techniques used to achieve maximum functioning and optimum adjustment for the patient and to prevent relapses or recurrences of illness; sometimes termed tertiary *prevention*.

Reich, Wilhelm (1897-1957) German *psychoanalyst* who emigrated to the United States in 1939; noted for his emphasis on the necessity of free expression of sexual *libido* during orgasm (orgone) as a cure for *neurosis*.

Reik, Theodor (1888-1969) *Psychoanalyst* and early follower of *Freud* who made valuable contributions to psychoanalysis on the subjects of religion, masochism, and therapeutic technique.

reinforcement The strengthening of a response by reward or avoidance of punishment. This process is central in *operant conditioning*.

relatedness Sense of sympathy and empathy with others.

REM latency The time lag between *sleep* onset (Stage 2 sleep) and the first REM period minus any awake time.

REM sleep Rapid eye movement *sleep*.

reminiscence A normal, universal process of life review in the elderly prompted in part by the realization of approaching death. The person reviews past life and conflicts and possibilities for their resolution. *Depression*, *anxiety*, regret, and despair may be present.

remission Abatement of an illness.

repetition compulsion In *psychoanalytic* theory, the impulse to reenact earlier emotional experiences. Considered by *Freud* more fundamental than the *pleasure principle*. According to *Jones*, "The blind impulse to repeat earlier experiences and situations quite irrespective of any advantage that doing so might bring from a pleasure-pain point of view."

repression A *defense mechanism*, operating *unconsciously*, that banishes unacceptable ideas, fantasies, *affects*, or impulses from *consciousness* or that keeps out of consciousness what has never been conscious. Although not subject to voluntary recall, the repressed material may emerge in disguised form. Often confused with the conscious mechanism of *suppression*.

reserpine An alkaloid used for treatment of hypertension and anxiety.

resident A physician who is in graduate training to qualify as a specialist in a particular field of medicine, such as *psychiatry*. The *American Board of Psychiatry and Neurology* requires four years of postgraduate training in an approved facility to qualify for board examination in psychiatry.

residential treatment facility See *halfway house*.

resistance One's *conscious* or *unconscious* psychologic defense against bringing *repressed* (unconscious) thoughts to light.

respondent conditioning (classical conditioning, Pavlovian conditioning) Elicitation of a response by a stimulus that normally does not elicit that response. The response is one that is mediated primarily by the *autonomic nervous system* (such as salivation or a change in heart rate). A previously neutral stimulus is repeatedly presented just before an unconditioned stimulus that normally elicits that response. When the response subsequently occurs in the presence of the previously neutral stimulus, it is called a conditioned response, and the previously neutral stimulus, a conditioned stimulus.

retardation See *mental retardation* and *psychomotor retardation*.

retrograde amnesia See *amnesia*.

retrospective falsification *Unconscious* distortion of past experiences to conform to present emotional needs.

ribonucleic acid (RNA) A chemical substance involved in cellular protein synthesis. Its structure is coded for by *DNA* (*deoxyribonucleic acid*). May play a role in *memory*.

right to refuse treatment See *Table of Legal Terms*.

rigidity In *psychiatry*, excessive resistance to change. See also *parkinsonism* and *extrapyramidal syndrome*.

ritual A repetitive activity, usually a distorted or stereotyped elaboration of some routine of daily life, employed to relieve *anxiety*. Most commonly seen in *obsessive compulsive neurosis* (see under *neurosis*).

Rogers, Carl R. (1902-1987) Psychologist, a founder of humanistic psychology and known for developing a client-centered approach to psychotherapy, which permits the patient to take the lead in the focus, pace, and direction of therapy; coined the term "self-actualization" to describe self-discovery and personal growth.

role A pattern of behavior a person acquires or adopts as influenced and expected by significant people in his milieu.

Rorschach test See *Table of Psychologic Tests*.

rumination In psychiatry, obsessive preoccupation with ideas and recollections; also rare eating disorder of early childhood consisting of a return of food from the stomach without nausea or retching. It leads to loss of weight, failure to thrive, interference with growth and development, and, in about 25% of cases, death.

Rush, Benjamin (1745-1813) Early American physician, a signer of the Declaration of Independence, and author of the first American book on *psychiatry* (1812). He is called the father of American psychiatry.

S

sadism Pleasure derived from inflicting physical or psychologic pain or abuse on others. The sexual significance of sadistic wishes or behavior may be *conscious* or *unconscious*. When necessary for sexual gratification, classifiable as a *paraphilia*.

sadomasochistic relationship Enjoyment of suffering by one person of an interacting couple with a complementary enjoyment in inflicting pain in the other.

satyriasis Pathologic or exaggerated sexual drive or excitement in the man. May be of psychologic or organic *etiology*. See also *nymphomania*.

schizoaffective disorder A depressive or manic *syndrome* that precedes or develops concurrently with *psychotic* symptoms incompatible with a mood disorder. Includes some *symptoms* characteristic of *schizophrenia* and other symptoms seen in *mood disorders*.

schizophrenia A large group of disorders, usually of *psychotic* proportion, manifested by characteristic disturbances of language and communication, thought, *perception*, *affect*, and behavior which last longer than six months. Thought disturbances are marked by alterations of concept formation that may lead to misinterpretation of reality, misperceptions, and sometimes to *delusions* and *hallucinations*. Mood changes include *ambivalence*, blunting, inappropriateness, and loss of *empathy* with others. Behavior may be withdrawn, *regressive*, and bizarre. The clinical picture is not explainable by any of the *organic mental disorders*. In the following list of recognized subtypes of schizophrenia, an asterisk (*) appears next to the official diagnostic terms in *DSM-III-R:*

acute Characterized by sudden onset of symptoms, often associated with confusion, perplexity, *ideas of reference*, emotional turmoil, excitement, *depression*, *fear*, or dreamlike *dissociation*. See also *schizophreniform disorder*.

catatonic* A marked psychomotor disturbance which may involve particular forms of *stupor*, rigidity, excitement, or posturing. Sometimes where there is a rapid alternation between the extremes of excitement and stupor, associated features include negativism, stereotypy, and *waxy flexibility*. *Mutism* is common.

childhood Schizophrenia appearing before puberty. Frequently manifested by *autism* and withdrawn behavior; failure to develop an *identity* separate from the mother's; general unevenness, gross immaturity, and inadequacy in development.

disorganized* **(hebephrenic)** Characterized by disorganized thinking, shallow and inappropriate *affect*, inappropriate giggling, silly and *regressive* behavior and mannerisms, and frequent *hypochondriacal* complaints. *Delusions* and *hallucinations* are usually bizarre and disorganized.

latent Clear *symptoms* of schizophrenia but no history of psychotic schizophrenic episodes. Sometimes designated as incipient, prepsychotic, pseudoneurotic, pseudopsychopathic, or borderline schizophrenia.

paranoid* Characterized by a persistence of or preoccupation with persecutory or grandiose *delusions*, or *hallucinations* with a persecutory or grandiose content. In addition, there may be delusions of jealousy.

process Attributed more to organic factors than to environmental ones; typically begins gradually, continues chronically, and progresses (either rapidly or slowly) to an irreversible *psychosis*. Contrast with *reactive schizophrenia*.

reactive Attributed primarily to strong predisposing and/or precipitating environmental factors; usually of rapid onset and brief duration, with the affected individual appearing well both before and after the schizophrenic episode. Differentiating this condition from process schizophrenia is generally considered more important in Europe than in this country. *Schizophreniform disorder* is conceptually similar.

residual* A condition manifested by persons with signs of schizophrenia who, following a psychotic schizophrenic episode, are no longer psychotic.

undifferentiated* A condition manifested by definite signs of schizophrenic thought, *affect*, and behavior that are of a sufficiently mixed or indefinite type that they defy classification into one of the other types of schizophrenia.

schizophreniform disorder Clinical features are the same as seen in *schizophrenia*, but the duration is less than six months but longer than one week. This disorder is believed to have different correlates than schizophrenia, including a better prognosis. See also *reactive schizophrenia*, under *schizophrenia* and *schizoaffective disorder*.

school phobia A term used when a child, usually in the early elementary grades, unexpectedly and strenuously refuses to attend school because of some irrational fear. The underlying *psychopathology* is believed to be an intense *separation anxiety* rooted in unresolved dependency ties. May occur in childhood *depression*.

schools of psychiatry The various theoretical frames of reference that influence and determine *psychiatrists'* formulations and methods of treatment. Most commonly the schools explain how psychiatric symptoms or disorders develop, how they interfere with functioning, and how and why they can be altered by therapeutic interventions. See also *Table of Schools in Psychiatry* for an arbitrary listing of schools and their founders or leading proponents.

scotoma A figurative blind spot in a person's psychologic awareness. Also, a *neurologic* term indicating a visual defect.

screen memory A *consciously* tolerable memory which serves as a cover for an associated memory that would be emotionally painful if recalled.

secondary gain The external gain derived from any illness, such as personal attention and service, monetary gains, disability benefits, and release from unpleasant responsibility. See also *primary gain*.

secondary process In *psychoanalytic* theory, mental activity and thinking characteristic of the *ego* and influenced by the demands of the environment. Characterized by organization, systematization, *intellectualization*, and similar processes leading to logical thought and action in adult life. See also *primary process* and *reality principle*.

sedative A broad term applied to any agent that quiets, calms, or allays excitement. The term is generally restricted to drugs that are not primarily used to achieve relief from *anxiety*. See also *Table of Drugs Used in Psychiatry*.

self The psychophysical total of a person, including both *conscious* and *unconscious* attributes.

self-fulfilling prophecy A distortion of an event or situation that eventually leads an individual to behave as he is expected to behave by others in his social setting.

self-help groups Troubled people with a common problem who collectively help each other by personal and group support. Examples are *Alcoholics Anonymous* (AA), Gamblers Anonymous (GA), and Narcotics Anonymous (NA).

senescence A chronologic period commonly referred to as old age; characterized by introspection, awareness of death, sense of legacy, and the possibilities of frailty, disability, dependency, and abandonment. Senescence is the result of physiologic, psychologic, and social forces.

senile dementia A chronic, progressive *dementia* associated with generalized atrophy of the brain with the death of neurons due to unknown causes, although there are several promising theories under study (e.g., autoimmunity, slow virus, cholinergic deficiency). It is not due to aging per se, but may be a late form of *Alzheimer's disease*. Deterioration may range from minimal to severe. It must be carefully separated from reversible brain syndrome, resulting from many causes. In *DSM-III-R*, it is listed as primary degenerative dementia, senile onset.

sensitivity group A group in which members strive to increase self-awareness and understanding of the group's dynamics, as distinct from treatments designed to ameliorate identified, individual, *ego-dystonic* emotional problems.

sensorium Synonymous with *consciousness*. Includes the special sensory perceptive powers and their central correlation and integration in the brain. A clear sensorium conveys the presence of a reasonably accurate memory together with *orientation* for time, place, and person. See also *mental status*.

sensory deprivation The experience of being cut off from usual external stimuli and the opportunity for perception. This may occur experimentally or accidentally in various ways. For example, the loss of hearing or eyesight, physical isolation, or some hospital confinements may lead to disorganized thinking, *delirium*, *depression*, *panic*, *delusions*, and *hallucinations*.

separation anxiety The *fear* and apprehension noted in infants when removed from the mother (or surrogate mother) or when approached by strangers. Most marked from sixth to tenth month. In later life, similar reactions may be caused by separation from significant persons or familiar surroundings.

separation-individuation Psychologic awareness of one's separateness, described by Margaret Mahler as a phase in the mother-child relationship that follows the symbiotic stage. In the separation-individuation stage, the child begins to perceive himself as distinct from the mother and develops a sense of individual identity and an image of the self as object. Mahler described four subphases of the process: differentiation, practicing, rapprochement (active approach toward the mother, replacing the relative obliviousness to her that prevailed during the practicing period), and separation-individuation proper (awareness of discrete identity, separateness, and individuality). See also *symbiosis*.

serotonin A *neurotransmitter* with an indole structure found both in peripheral ganglia and in the *central nervous system*. Its transmitter functions in the central nervous system are less clearly demonstrable than in the gastrointestinal tract. It is implicated indirectly in the psychobiology of *depression*. See also *biogenic amines*.

serum levels See *blood levels*.

sexual deviation See *paraphilia*.

sexual disorders A *DSM-III-R* term for *psychosexual dysfunction*.

sexual drive One of the two primal drives (the other is aggressive drive) according to *Freud*'s dual-instinct theory.

shaman A healer whose ability comes from trancelike or supernatural experiences.

shame An *emotion* resulting from the failure to live up to self-expectations. See also *guilt* and *superego*.

shaping Reinforcement of responses in the patient's repertoire that increasingly approximate sought-after behavior.

shell shock Term used in World War I to designate a wide variety of *mental disorders* presumably due to combat experience. See also *combat fatigue*.

shock treatment An inaccurate term often used to refer to *electroconvulsive treatment*.

short-term memory The recognition, recall, and reproduction of perceived material 10 seconds or longer after initial presentation See also *immediate memory*.

sibling A full brother or sister.

sibling rivalry The competition between *siblings* for the love of a parent or for other recognition or gain.

"sick role" An identity adopted by an individual as a "patient" that specifies a set of expected behaviors, usually dependent.

side effect A drug response that accompanies the principal response for which a medication is taken. Most side effects are undesirable yet cause only minor annoyances; others may cause serious problems.

sign Objective evidence of disease or disorder. See also *symptom*.

signal anxiety Attenuated *anxiety* that functions as an early warning system for the *ego*. It derives from the normal capacity to anticipate a potentially dangerous situation and react to it by deploying emergency defenses before it becomes intense. Signal anxiety may progress to a full-fledged anxiety attack or even to a *panic* state if the early warning is not heeded or if available defenses prove insufficient. A situation becomes traumatic when the influx of stimuli is too great for the *psyche* to master or discharge.

simple phobia See *phobic neurosis* under *neurosis*.

Skinner, Burrhus Frederic (1904-   ) American *psychologist* noted for his research and writings on *operant conditioning*. Many of the procedures of *behavior therapy* are based on laboratory research by Skinner and his students.

sleep The recurring period of relative physical and psychologic disengagement from one's environment accompanied by characteristic EEG (electroencephalogram) findings and divisible into two categories: non-rapid eye movement (NREM) sleep, also known as orthodox or synchronized (S) sleep; and rapid eye movement (REM) sleep, also referred to as paradoxical or desynchronized (D) sleep. Dreaming sleep is another, though less accurate, term for REM sleep. Four stages of NREM-sleep based on EEG findings are stage 1, occurring immediately after sleep begins, with a pattern of low amplitude and fast frequency; stage 2, having characteristic waves of 12-16 cycles per second known as sleep spindles; stages 3 and 4, having progressive further slowing of frequency and increase in amplitude of the wave forms.

Over a period of 90 minutes after the beginning of sleep, a person has progressed through the 4 stages of NREM sleep and emerges from them into the first period of REM sleep. REM sleep is associated with dreaming, and brief cycles (20-30 minutes) of this sleep recur about every 90 minutes throughout the night. Coordinated rapid eye movements give this type of sleep its name. Sleep patterns vary with age, state of health, medication, and psychologic state. See also *sleep terror disorder* and *somnambulism*.

sleep terror disorder Condition occurring in stage 4 *sleep* manifested by *panic*, confusion, and poor recall for the event. Contrast with *nightmares*.

sleepwalking disorder See *somnambulism*.

social adaption The ability to live and express oneself according to society's restrictions and cultural demands.

social breakdown syndrome The concept that some psychiatric symptomatology is a result of treatment conditions and inadequate facilities and not a part of the primary illness. Factors bringing about the condition are social labeling, learning the role of the chronically sick, atrophy of work and social skills, and *identification* with the sick. See also *rehabilitation*.

social phobia See *phobic neurosis* under *neurosis*.

social psychiatry The field of *psychiatry* concerned with the cultural, ecologic, and sociologic factors that engender, precipitate, intensify, prolong, or otherwise complicate maladaptive patterns of behavior and their treatment.

social work The use of community resources and the *conscious* adaptive capacities of individuals and groups to better their adjustment to their environment.

social worker, psychiatric A skilled professional, usually with a M.S.W., trained in social work who works with psychiatrists usually in an institutional setting. Psychiatric social workers also carry out individual, family, and group psychotherapy.

socialization The process by which society integrates the person and the way he learns to become a functioning member of that society. See also *sociology*.

sociobiology The study of the evolution of social behavior. Its roots lie in evolutionary biology, *ethology*, and comparative *psychology*.

sociology The study of the governing principles and development of social organization and the group behavior of people, in contrast to individual behavior. It overlaps to some extent with *cultural anthropology*. See also *alienation* and *socialization*.

sociometry The science of assessing the interpersonal psychologic structure of a group or society.

sociopath An unofficial term for *antisocial personality*. See under *personality disorders*.

sociotherapy Any treatment in which emphasis is on socioenvironmental and interpersonal rather than on *intrapsychic* factors, as in the *therapeutic community*. In most forms of sociotherapy, peer acceptance is an important element, typically achieved through confrontation by the group when peer expectations are not met.

sodomy Anal intercourse. Legally, the term may include other types of perversion such as *bestiality*. See also *paraphilia*.

soma The body.

somatic therapy In *psychiatry*, the biologic treatment of mental disorders (e.g., *electroconvulsive therapy*, *psychopharmacologic* treatment). Contrast with *psychotherapy*.

somatization disorder Multiple, recurrent, and long-term somatic complaints which are apparently not due to any physical disorder. The complaints begin before the age of 30 and have a chronic but fluctuating course. In *DSM-III-R*, it is classified as one of the *somatoform disorders*. Also known as *Briquet's syndrome*.

somatoform disorders A group of disorders with symptoms suggesting physical disorders but without demonstrable organic findings to explain the symptoms. There is positive evidence, or a strong presumption, that the symptoms are linked to psychologic factors or *conflicts*. In *DSM-III-R*, this category includes *somatization disorder, conversion disorder, hypochondriasis,* and body dysmorphic disorder.

somnambulism A *sleep* disorder in which motor acts (such as walking) are performed. In *DSM-III-R*, it is called sleepwalking disorder.

speech disturbance Any disorder of verbal communication that is not due to faulty innervation of speech muscles or organs of articulation. The term includes many language and *learning disabilities*. Contrast with *agraphia, aphasia,* and *apraxia* in *Table of Neurologic Deficits*. See also *amimia* and *dyslexia*.

standard deviation See *Table of Research Terms*.

Stanford-Binet Intelligence Scale See *Table of Psychologic Tests*.

status epilepticus Continuous epileptic seizures. See *epilepsy*.

stereotypy Persistent, mechanical repetition of speech or motor activity. observed in *schizophrenia*.

stimulants See *Table of Drugs Used in Psychiatry*.

Stockholm syndrome A syndrome in which hostages identify with, and have sympathy for, their captors on whom they are dependent for survival. Not uncommonly seen in terrorist-hostage situations.

street drugs See *Table of Commonly Abused Drugs*.

strephosymbolia A tendency to reverse letters and words in reading and writing. Seen in *learning disability*.

stress reaction An acute, maladaptive emotional response to industrial, domestic, civilian or military disasters, and other calamitous life situations; it may also be chronic, as seen in some Vietnam veterans.

stroke Cerebrovascular accident (CVA); gross cerebral hemorrhage or softening of the brain following hemorrhage, thrombosis, or embolism of the cerebral arteries. *Symptoms* may include *coma*, paralysis (particularly on one side of the body), *convulsions*, *aphasia*, and other neurologic signs determined by the location of the lesion.

stupor A state in which a person does not react to or is unaware of the surroundings. Due to neurologic as well as psychiatric disorders. In catatonic stupor, the unawareness is more apparent than real. See also *catatonia*.

subconscious Obsolete term. Formerly used to include the *preconscious* (what can be recalled with effort) and the *unconscious*.

sublimation A *defense mechanism*, operating *unconsciously*, by which *instinctual drives, consciously* unacceptable, are diverted into personally and socially acceptable channels.

substance abuse See *drug dependence*.

substitution A *defense mechanism*, operating *unconsciously*, by which an unattainable or unacceptable goal, *emotion*, or object is replaced by one that is more attainable or acceptable.

succinylcholine A drug used intravenously in *anesthesia* as a skeletal muscle relaxant. Also used prior to *electroconvulsive treatment* to minimize the possibility of complications.

suggestibility Uncritical compliance or acceptance of an idea, belief, or attribute.

suggestion The process of influencing a patient to accept an idea, belief, or attitude suggested by the therapist. See also *hypnosis*.

suicide Taking of one's own life.

suicide, cluster See *cluster suicides*.

Sullivan, Harry Stack (1892-1949) American *psychiatrist* and *psychoanalyst* known for his research in the *psychotherapy* of *schizophrenia* and for his view of complex interpersonal relationships as the basis of personality development.

superego In *psychoanalytic* theory, that part of the *personality* structure associated with ethics, standards, and self-criticism. It is formed by *identification* with important and esteemed persons in early life, particularly parents. The supposed or actual wishes of these significant persons are taken over as part of the child's own standards to help form the *conscience*. See also *ego*, *id*, *guilt*, and *shame*.

supportive psychotherapy A type of *psychotherapy* that aims to reinforce a patient's defenses and help suppress disturbing psychologic material. Supportive psychotherapy utilizes such measures as inspiration, reassurance, suggestion, persuasion, counseling, and reeducation. It avoids probing the patient's emotional conflicts in depth. See also *psychotherapy*.

suppression The *conscious* effort to control and conceal unacceptable impulses, thoughts, feelings, or acts.

symbiosis A mutually reinforcing relationship between two persons who are dependent on each other; a normal characteristic of the relationship between the mother and infant child.

symbiotic psychosis A condition seen in two- to four-year-old children with an abnormal relationship to a mothering figure. The *psychosis* is characterized by intense *separation anxiety*, severe *regression*, giving up of useful speech, and *autism*.

symbolization A general mechanism in all human thinking by which some mental representation comes to stand for some other thing, class of things, or attribute of something. This mechanism underlies dream formation and some *symptoms*, such as conversion reactions, *obsessions,* and compulsions. The link between the latent meaning of the symptom and the symbol is usually *unconscious.*

sympathetic nervous system The part of the *autonomic nervous system* that responds to dangerous or threatening situations by preparing a person physiologically for "fight or flight." See also *parasympathetic nervous system.*

sympathy A feeling or capacity for sharing in the interests or concerns of another. May arise when there is no emotional attachment to the person toward whom one is sympathetic, since the feelings of the sympathetic person remain essentially internal. Contrast with *empathy.*

symptom A specific manifestation of a patient's condition indicative of an abnormal physical or mental state; a subjective perception of illness.

symptomatic psychoses See *organic mental disorder.*

synapse The gap between the membrane of one nerve cell and the membrane of another. The synapse is the point at which the transmission of nerve impulses occurs.

syndrome A configuration of *symptoms* that occur together and constitute a recognizable condition.

syntaxic mode The mode of perception that forms whole, logical, coherent pictures of reality that can be validated by others.

syphilis A sexually transmitted venereal disease, which, if untreated, may lead to *central nervous system* deterioration with *psychotic* manifestations in its later stages. See also *general paralysis*.

systematic desensitization (desensitization) A *behavior therapy* procedure widely used to modify behaviors associated with *phobias*. The procedure involves the construction of a hierarchy of *anxiety*-producing stimuli by the subject, and gradual presentation of the stimuli until they no longer produce anxiety. See also *reciprocal inhibition*.

T

taboo Prohibitions and restrictions interwoven in the culture.

talion law or principle A primitive, unrealistic belief, usually *unconscious*, conforming to the Biblical injunction of an "eye for an eye and a tooth for a tooth." In *psychoanalysis*, the concept and fear that all injury, actual or intended, will be punished in kind.

tangentiality Replying to a question in an oblique or irrelevant way. Compare with *circumstantiality*.

Tarasoff decision A California court decision which essentially imposes a duty on the therapist to warn the appropriate person or persons when he becomes aware that his patient may present a risk of harm to a specific person or persons.

tardive dyskinesia Literally, "late-appearing abnormal movements"; a variable complex of choreiform or athetoid movements developing in patients exposed to antipsychotic drugs. Typical movements include tongue-writhing or protrusion, chewing, lip-puckering, choreiform finger movements, toe and ankle movements, leg-jiggling, or movements of neck, trunk, and pelvis. These movements may be either mild or severe and may occur singly or in many combinations and permutations. See also antipsychotic drugs in *Table of Drugs Used in Psychiatry*.

TAT (Thematic Apperception Test) See *Table of Psychologic Tests*.

telepathy Communication of thought from one person to another without the intervention of physical means. See also *extrasensory perception, parapsychology*.

temperament Constitutional predisposition to react in a particular way to stimuli.

temporal lobe epilepsy Complex partial seizures; psychomotor epilepsy. See *epilepsy*.

testamentary capacity See *Table of Legal Terms*.

thanatology The study of death and dying, emphasizing therapeutic interventions with the dying and their survivors.

therapeutic community A term of British origin, now widely used, for a specially structured mental hospital milieu that encourages patients to function within the range of social norms.

therapeutic window The well-defined range of *blood levels* associated with optimal clinical response to anti-depressant drugs, such as nortriptyline. Levels above or below that range are associated with a poor response.

thioxanthene derivatives See *Table of Drugs Used in Psychiatry*.

third ear (the) Literally, listening with "the third ear," that is, the utilization of intuition, sensitivity, and aware-ness of subliminal cues to interpret clinical observations of patients in therapy.

third party payer Any organization (public or private) that pays or insures health or medical expenses on be-half of beneficiaries or recipients. Examples are Blue Cross and Blue Shield, *Medicare*, *Medicaid*, and com-mercial insurance companies.

thought disorder A disturbance of speech, communica-tion, or content of thought, such as *delusions*, *ideas of reference*, poverty of thought, *flight of ideas*, *persevera-tion*, *loosening of associations*, etc. A thought disorder can be caused by a functional emotional disorder or an organic condition. A formal thought disorder is a distur-bance in the form of thought rather than the content of thought, e.g., *loosening of associations*.

tic An intermittent, involuntary, spasmodic movement of a group of muscles, often without a demonstrable exter-nal stimulus. A tic may be an expression of an emotional conflict or the result of *neurologic* disease.

token economy A system involving the application of the principles and procedures of *operant conditioning* to the management of a social setting such as a ward, classroom, or halfway house. Tokens are given contingent on completion of specified activities and are exchangeable for goods or privileges desired by the patient.

tomography Imaging of serial planes ("cuts") through an anatomical structure. See also *brain imaging*.

Tourette's syndrome See *Gilles de la Tourette syndrome*.

toxic psychosis An *organic mental disorder* caused by the poisonous effect of chemicals or drugs.

toxicity The capacity of a drug to damage body tissue or seriously impair body functions.

trance A state of focused attention and diminished sensory and motor activity seen in *hypnosis, hysterical neurosis, dissociative types* (see under *neurosis*), and ecstatic religious states.

tranquilizer A drug that decreases *anxiety* and *agitation*. Preferred terms are antianxiety and antipsychotic drugs. See also *Table of Drugs Used in Psychiatry*.

transactional analysis A *psychodynamic psychotherapy* based on role theory that attempts to understand the interplay between therapist and patient and ultimately between the patient and external reality. See also *Table of Schools of Psychiatry*.

transcultural psychiatry See *cross-cultural psychiatry*.

transference The *unconscious* assignment to others of feelings and attitudes that were originally associated with important figures (parents, *siblings*, etc.) in one's early life. The transference relationship follows the pattern of its prototype. The *psychiatrist* utilizes this phenomenon as a therapeutic tool to help the patient understand emotional problems and their origins. In the patient-physician relationship, the transference may be negative (hostile) or positive (affectionate). See also *countertransference* and *parataxic distortion*.

transsexual A disturbance of *gender identity* in which the person feels a life-long discomfort with his or her own sex and a compelling desire to be of the opposite sex.

transvestism Sexual pleasure derived from dressing or masquerading in the clothing of the opposite sex, with the strong wish to appear as a member of the opposite sex. The sexual origins of transvestism may be *unconscious*.

trauma, psychic An *intrapsychic* event brought on by submission to an anticipated danger. The acute *syndrome* is characterized by psychologic shock; helplessness; numbness of feelings; disturbances of speech, eating, and sleeping (nightmares); and social withdrawal. Persistence of the helpless state may result in death. The long-term effects are usually persistent *narcissistic* preoccupation; *somatic* concerns; depressive and *anxiety* symptoms; and fear of being further victimized.

traumatic neurosis See *posttraumatic stress disorder*.

trichotillomania An impulse disorder. See also under -*mania*.

tricyclic antidepressants See *Table of Drugs Used in Psychiatry*.

trisomy The presence of three *chromosomes* instead of the two that normally represent each potential set of chromosomes. This can result in a *developmental disability*. An example of trisomy is *Down's syndrome*.

Tuke, William (1732-1822) English Quaker layman who pioneered in treating psychiatric patients without using physical restraints.

Turner's syndrome A *chromosomal* defect in women with a karyotype of XO and 45 chromosomes rather than the usual 46. Clinical features of this disorder are small stature, webbed neck, abnormal ovarian development, and sometimes *mental retardation*.

twin research A powerful method of investigating the relative degree of phenotypic variance that can be attributed to genetic factors and to transmissible and nontransmissible environmental factors. For example, the dissimilarities between *monozygotic* twins are compared with the behavioral variations occurring in nontwin siblings or *dizygotic* twins.

type A personality A *temperament* characterized by excessive drive, competitiveness, a sense of time urgency, impatience, unrealistic ambition, and need for control. Believed to be associated with a high incidence of coronary artery disease.

type B personality A *temperament* characterized by a relaxed, easy-going demeanor; less time-bound and competitive than the type A *personality*.

tyramine A sympathomimetic amine that acts by displacing stored transmitter from adrenergic axonal terminals; a constituent of many foods such as flat beans, cheese, red wine, etc., which are forbidden when using *monoamine oxidase inhibitors* because of *hypertensive crisis*.

U

ultradian rhythms See *biologic rhythms*.

unconscious That part of the mind or mental functioning of which the content is only rarely subject to awareness. It is a repository for data that have never been *conscious* (primary *repression*) or that may have become conscious briefly and later repressed (secondary *repression*).

undoing A *defense mechanism*, operating *unconsciously*, in which something unacceptable and already done is symbolically *acted out* in reverse, usually repetitiously, in the hope of relieving *anxiety*. See also *obsessive compulsive neurosis* under *neurosis*.

unipolar psychoses Recurrent major *depressions*. See *major affective disorders*.

utilization review committee A committee of physicians and other clinical staff formed in a hospital to review the quality of services rendered, as well as the effective and appropriate use of facilities. See also *peer review organization*.

V

variance See *Table of Research Terms*.

vegetative nervous system Obsolete term for the *autonomic nervous system*.

verbigeration Stereotyped and seemingly meaningless repetition of words or sentences. See also *perseveration*.

vertigo A sensation that the external world is spinning around; a symptom of vestibular dysfunction.

vitamin therapy See *orthomolecular treatment*.

voluntary admission See *commitment*.

voyeurism Sexually motivated and often compulsive interest in watching or looking at others, particularly at genitals. A "Peeping Tom" represents a pathologic expression of voyeurism. See also *compulsion*.

W

Wagner von Jauregg, Julius (1857-1940) Austrian *psychiatrist* who won the Nobel Prize in 1927 for research in using malaria inoculation and other artificially induced fevers in treating syphilis of the *central nervous system*.

Watson, John B. (1878-1958) American *psychologist*; the founder of the behaviorism school of *psychology*.

waxy flexibility See *cerea flexibilitas*.

Wechsler Adult Intelligence Scale (WAIS) See *Table of Psychologic Tests*.

Wednesday Evening Society A group of Freud's followers and students who formed the basis of the Vienna Psychoanalytic Society.

weekend hospitalization See *partial hospitalization*.

Wernicke-Korsakoff syndrome A disease of *central nervous system* metabolism due to a lack of vitamin B1 (thiamine) seen in chronic *alcoholism*. Wernicke's disease features irregularities of *eye* movements, incoordination, impaired thinking, and often sensorimotor deficits. *Korsakoff's psychosis* is characterized by *confabulation* and, more importantly, by a short-term, but not immediate, disturbance that leads to gross impairment in memory and learning. Wernicke's disease and Korsakoff's psychosis begin suddenly and are often found in the same person simultaneously. See also *alcoholic psychosis*.

Weyer, Johann (circa 1530) Dutch physician who was one of the first to devote his major interest to psychiatric disorders. Regarded by some as the founder of modern *psychiatry*.

White, William Alanson (1870-1937) American *psychiatrist* famous for his early support of *psychoanalysis* and his contributions to *forensic psychiatry*.

windigo See *culture-specific syndromes*.

withdrawal A pathologic retreat from people or the world of reality, often seen in *schizophrenia*.

withdrawal symptoms Physical and mental effects of withdrawing addictive substances from patients who have become habituated to them. The physical symptoms may include vomiting, tremors, abdominal pain, *delirium*, and *convulsions*. See also *addiction* and *delirium tremens*.

word salad A mixture of words and phrases that lack comprehensive meaning or logical coherence, commonly seen in *schizophrenic* states.

word-blindness See *learning disability*.

working through Exploration of a problem by patient and therapist until a satisfactory solution has been found or until a *symptom* has been traced to its *unconscious* sources.

World Psychiatric Association (WPA) A nongovernmental organization composed of about 75 member societies from as many countries. Its headquarters are based in the home country of its secretariat.

X

x-linkage Mode of genetic transmission in which a tract or *gene* is linked to the X chromosome. Has been implicated in some cases of *bipolar disorder*.

xenophobia See under *phobia*.

Z

zeitgeist The general intellectual and cultural climate of taste characteristic of an era.

zygosity (dizygotic and **monozygotic)** See *Table of Research Terms*.

REFERENCES

Diagnostic and Statistical Manual of Mental Disorders, 3rd Edition, Revised. American Psychiatric Association, Washington, DC, 1987.

Psychiatric Dictionary, 5th Edition, R.J. Campbell, Oxford University Press, New York, 1981.

LIST OF COMMONLY USED ABBREVIATIONS

AA Alcoholics Anonymous

AAAS American Association for the Advancement of Science

AABA American Anorexia/Bulimia Association, Inc.

AACAP American Academy of Child and Adolescent Psychiatry

AACDP American Association of Chairmen of Departments of Psychiatry

AACMHP American Association of Community Mental Health Center Psychiatrists

AACP American Academy of Clinical Psychiatrists

AACP American Academy for Child Psychoanalysts

AADPRT American Association of Directors of Psychiatric Residency Training, Inc.

AAFP American Academy of Family Physicians

AAGP American Association for Geriatric Psychiatry

AAGHP American Association of General Hospital Psychiatrists

AAMC Association of American Medical Colleges

AAMD American Association on Mental Deficiency

AAMFT American Association for Marriage and Family Therapy

AAMR American Academy on Mental Retardation

177

AAN American Academy of Neurology

AANP American Association of Neuropathologists

AAP American Academy of Psychoanalysis

AAP American Academy of Psychotherapists

AAP Association for the Advancement of Psychotherapy

AAP Association for Academic Psychiatry

AAP Association for the Advancement of Psychoanalysis

AAPA American Association of Psychiatric Administrators

AAPAA American Association of Psychiatrists in Alcoholism and the Addictions

AAPC American Association of Pastoral Counselors

AAPH American Association for Partial Hospitalization

AAPL American Academy of Psychiatry and the Law

AAPSC American Association of Psychiatric Services for Children

AAPT Association for the Advancement of Psychotherapy

AAS American Association of Suicidology

AASP American Association for Social Psychiatry

AATA American Art Therapy Association

ABFP American Board of Forensic Psychiatry

ABMS American Board of Medical Specialties

ABPN *American Board of Psychiatry and Neurology*

ACMHA American College of Mental Health Administration

ACMPD American Council on Marijuana and Other Psychoactive Drugs

ACNP American College of Neuropsychiatrists

ACNPP American College of Neuropsychopharmacology

ACP American College of Psychiatrists

ACP American College of Physicians

ACP Association for Child Psychoanalysis

ACPA American College of Psychoanalysts

ACTH Adrenocorticotropic hormone

AD *Alzheimer's* disease

ADAMHA *Alcohol, Drug Abuse, and Mental Health Administration*

ADD *attention deficit disorder (DSM-III-R)*

ADMSEP Association of Directors of Medical Student Education in Psychiatry

ADPANA Alcohol and Drug Problems Association of North America

ADRDA *Alzheimer's Disease* and Related Disorders Association

AFCR American Federation for Clinical Research

AFTA American Family Therapy Association

AGS American Geriatrics Society

AGPTA American Group Psychotherapy Association

AHA American Hospital Association

AHCA American Health Care Association

AIBS American Institute of Biological Sciences

AIDS acquired immune deficiency syndrome *(AIDS)*

AIPP American Institute for Psychotherapy and Psychoanalysis

AIS American Institute of Stress

AJP *American Journal of Psychiatry*

AMA against medical advice

AMA American Medical Association

AMERSA Association for Medical Education and Research in Substance Abuse

AMHA Association of Mental Health Administrators

AMHC Association of Mental Health Clergy

AMHCA American Mental Health Counselors Association

AMHF American Mental Health Fund

AMHL Association of Mental Health Librarians

AMSA American Medical Society on Alcoholism

AMSA American Medical Student Association

AMWA American Medical Women's Association

ANA American Neurologic Association

ANA American Nurses' Association

ANFMP Association of Nervous and Former Mental Patients (Recovery, Inc.)

ANS *autonomic nervous system*

AOA American Orthopsychiatric Association

AOTA American Occupational Therapy Association

APA *American Psychiatric Association*

APA American Psychoanalytic Association

APA American Psychological Association

APAL Asociacion Psiquitrica de America Latina

APM Academy of Psychosomatic Medicine

APPA American Psychopathological Association

APPI American Psychiatric Press, Inc.

APPM Association for Psychoanalytic and Psychosomatic Medicine

APS American Psychosomatic Society, Inc.

ARC Association for Retarded Citizens

ARMH Academy of Religion and Mental Health

ARNMD Association for Research in Nervous and Mental Disease

ASA American Schizophrenia Association

ASAP American Society for Adolescent Psychiatry

ASF American Schizophrenia Foundation

ASGPP American Society of Group Psychotherapy and Psychodrama

ASLM American Society of Law and Medicine

ASPP American Society of Psychoanalytic Physicians

AWA away without authorization

BASH Bulimia Anorexia Self-Help, Inc.

BEAM *brain electrical activity mapping*

B.I.D. twice a day

BIS Brain Information Service

BMA British Medical Association

BRF Brain Research Foundation

BTRS Behavior Therapy and Research Society

CA Cocaine Anonymous

CAT *Children's Apperception Test*

CAT *computerized axial tomography*

CBT cognitive behavioral therapy

CMA Canadian Medical Association

CME *continuing medical education*

CMHA Canadian Mental Health Association

CMHC *community mental health center*

CMSS Council of Medical Specialty Societies

CNS *central nervous system*

CPA Canadian Psychiatric Association

CPA Caribbean Psychiatric Association

CPDD Committee on Problems of Drug Dependence

CPT Current Procedural Terminology (AMA)

CRF corticotropic-releasing factor

CSF cerebrospinal fluid

CT *computerized axial tomography*

CVA cerebrovascular accident; *stroke*

CWLA Child Welfare League of America, Inc.

DBH dopamine beta-hydroxylase

DHHS Department of *Health and Human Services*

DMH Department of Mental Health/Department of Mental Hygiene

DNA *deoxyribonucleic acid*

DOV discharged on visit

DRG *diagnostic related group*

DSM *Diagnostic and Statistical Manual of Mental Disorders*

DSM-III-R *Diagnostic and Statistical Manual of Mental Disorders, Third Edition, Revised*

DST Dexamethasone Suppression Test

DTs *delirium tremens*

ECA epidemiologic catchment area

ECFMG Educational Commission for Foreign Medical Graduates

ECT *electroconvulsive treatment*

EE expressed emotion

EEG *electroencephalogram*

EFA Epilepsy Foundation of America

EKG electrocardiogram; also ECG

EMG *electromyogram*

EPRA Eastern Psychiatric Research Association

ESP *extrasensory perception*

EST *electroconvulsive treatment*

FDA *Food and Drug Administration*

FDMD Foundation for Depression and Manic Depression

GA Gamblers Anonymous

GAP Group for the Advancement of Psychiatry

GSR *galvanic skin response*

H&CP *Hospital and Community Psychiatry* (APA)

HIBR Huxley Institute for Biosocial Research

HMO *health maintenance organization*

HRS Hamilton Rating Scale

HLTV-III virus involved in *AIDS*

IACPA Inter-American Council of Psychiatric Associations

IALMH International Academy of Law and Mental Health

IASP International Association for Suicide Prevention

IASSMD International Association for the Scientific Study of Mental Deficiency

ICAMI/WRAPD International Committee Against Mental Illness and World Rehabilitation Association for the Psycho-Socially Disabled

ICD *International Classification of Diseases*

ICPM International College of Psychosomatic Medicine

ICSW International Council on Social Welfare

IFMP International Federation for Medical Psychotherapy

IFPS International Federation of Psychoanalytic Societies

IM/NAS Institute of Medicine/National Academy of Sciences

IND investigational new drug

IPAAE International Psychiatric Association for the Advancement of Electrotherapy

IPT interpersonal therapy

IQ *intelligence quotient*

ITAA International Transactional Analysis Association

JCAH *Joint Commission on Accreditation of Hospitals*

JCMHC *Joint Commission on Mental Health of Children*

JCMIH *Joint Commission on Mental Illness and Health*

JCPA Joint Commission on Public Affairs (APA)

LP *lumbar puncture*

LSD lysergic acid diethylamide *(LSD)*

MAOI *monoamine oxidase inhibitor*

MBD *minimal brain dysfunction*

MDI *manic depressive illness*

MHA Mental Health Association

MMPI Minnesota Multiphasic Personality Inventory (See *Table of Psychologic Tests)*

MRAA Mental Retardation Association of America

MRI *magnetic resonance imaging*

NA Narcotics Anonymous

NADS National Association for Down's Syndrome

NAIL Neurotics Anonymous International Liaison

NAMH National Association for Mental Health

NAMI *National Alliance for the Mentally Ill*

NAMT National Association for Music Therapy

NANAD National Association of Anorexia and Associated Disorders

NAPPH National Association of Private Psychiatric Hospitals

NARC National Association for Retarded Citizens

NARSD National Alliance for Research on Schizophrenia and Depression

NASMHPD National Association of State Mental Health Program Directors

NASMHRI National Association of State Mental Health Research Institutes

NASW National Association of Social Workers

NAVACP National Association of Veterans Administration Chiefs of Psychiatry

NBME National Board of Medical Examiners

NCA National Council on the Aging

NCAI National Council on Alcoholism, Inc.

NCCMHC National Council of Community Mental Health Centers

NCD National Council on Drugs

NDMDA National Depressive and Manic-Depressive Association

NGCP National Guild of Catholic Psychiatrists

NHC National Health Council

NIA National Institute on Aging

NIAAA National Institute on Alcohol Abuse and Alcoholism (see *Alcohol, Drug Abuse, and Mental Health Administration*)

NIDA National Institute on Drug Abuse (see *Alcohol, Drug Abuse and Mental Health Administration*)

NIMH National Institute of Mental Health (see *Alcohol, Drug Abuse, and Mental Health Administration*)

NLN National League for Nursing

NMA National Medical Association

NMHA *National Mental Health Association*

NMHF National Mental Health Foundation

NMS *neuroleptic malignant syndrome*

NOMIC National Organization for Mentally Ill Children

NRA National Rehabilitation Association

NRC National Research Council

NREM non-rapid eye movement (see *sleep*)

NSAC National Society for Autistic Children

NSF National Science Foundation

OBD organic brain disease

OBS *organic brain syndrome*

PCMH Public Committee on Mental Health

PDR Physician's Desk Reference

PET *positron emission tomography*

PKU *phenylketonuria*

PPA Philippine Psychiatrists of America

PSR Physicians for Social Responsibility

PSRO *professional standards review organization*

QID four times a day

RANZCP Royal Australian and New Zealand College of Psychiatrists

REM rapid *eye* movement (*see sleep*)

RCP Royal College of Psychiatrists

RCPSC Royal College of Physicians and Surgeons of Canada

RNA *ribonucleic acid*

RSM Royal Society of Medicine

SA Schizophrenics Anonymous

SAI Schizophrenics Anonymous International

SADS seasonal affective disorder syndrome

SBM Society of Behavioral Medicine

SBP Society of Biological Psychiatry

SDAT *senile dementia, Alzheimer* type

SIECUS Sex Information and Education Council of the U.S.

SNS Society for Neuroscience

SPCP Society of Professors of Child Psychiatry

SMA Southern Medical Association

SPA Southern Psychiatric Association

SRS Sleep Research Society

SSI/SSDI Social Security Insurance/Social Security Disability Insurance

TIA transient ischemic attack

TID three times a day

TM transcendental meditation

TRH thyrotropin releasing hormone test

USPHS U.S. Public Health Service

VA Veterans Administration

WASP World Association for Social Psychiatry

WFMH World Federation for Mental Health

WHO World Health Organization

WMA World Medical Association

WPA *World Psychiatric Association*

TABLE OF COMMONLY ABUSED DRUGS

Class	Trade Name* (or Source)	Street Names
Opioids		
morphine	morphine sulfate	dope, M, Miss Emma, morpho, white stuff
heroin	none	H, junk, skag, smack, boy, hard stuff, horse
hydromorphone	Dilaudid	DL's
oxymorphone	Numorphan	blues
oxycodone	Percodan, Percocet	Percs
meperidine	Demerol	
methadone hydrochloride	Dolophine	dollys, done
pentazocine	Talwin	
tincture of opium	paregoric	PG, licorice
cough preparations with codeine	Elixir terpin hydrate	schoolboy, blue velvet
	Robitussin A-C	
hydrocodone	Hycodan	Robby
Non-narcotic Analgesic		
propoxyphene	Darvon	
Benzodiazepines		
diazepam	Valium	
chlordiazepoxide	Librium	
alprazolam	Xanax	
oxazepam	Serax	
lorazepam	Ativan	
Barbiturates		
secobarbital	Seconal	barbs, candy, dolls, goofers, peanuts, sleeping pill
amobarbital	Amytal	pink lady, red devils, red, seccy, pinks
pentobarbital	Nembutal	blue angels, bluebirds, blue devils, blues, lilly
phenobarbital	Luminal	nebbies, yellow bullets, yellow dolls
		phennies, purple hearts
amobarbital/secobarbital	Tuinal	Christmas trees, double-trouble, rainbows, tooies

Other Sedative-Hypnotics

methaqualone	Quaalude	sopors, ludes
gluthethimide	Doriden	CIBA's, packs (with codeine)
methyrpylon	Noludar	

Central Nervous System Stimulants

ethchlorvynol	Placidyl	
chloral hydrate	Noctec	
paraldehyde	Paral	
meprobamate	Miltown	
scopolamine	Sominex	truth serum
cocaine hydrochloride	cocaine	coke, blow, toot, girl
cocaine freebase		crack, rock, base
d, dl amphetamine	Biphetamine	black beauties
amphetamine sulfate	Benzedrine	A's, beans, bennies, cartwheels, crossroads, jelly beans, hearts, peaches, whites
amphetamine sulfate/ amobarbital	Dexamyl	greenies
dextroamphetamine sulfate	Dexedrine	brownies, Christmas trees, dexies, hearts, wakeups
methamphetamine hydrochloride	Methedrine	bombit, crank, crystal, meth, speed

Drugs with Hallucinogenic Properties

d lysergic acid diethylamide	synthetic derivative (ergot fungus)	acid, pink wedges, sandos, sugar cubes
psilocin/psilocybin	mushroom (psilocybe mexicana)	business man's acid, magic mushroom
dimethyltryptamine (DMT)	synthetic	DMT, DET, DPT
morning glory seeds	birdweed (rivea corymbosa)	flower power, heavenly blue, pearly gates
mescaline	peyote cactus	barf tea, big chief, buttons, cactus, mesc

*Many of these drugs are sold under a variety of trade names; only a single popular example is used for each.

Class	Trade Name* (or Source)	Street Names
Drugs with Hallucinogenic Properties (cont.)		
methyldimethoxy-amphetamine (DOM)	synthetic (derivative)	STP
myristicin	nutmeg	MMDA
muscarine	mushroom *(amanita muscaria)*	fly
phencyclidine		angel dust, dust, PCP
Tetrahydrocannabinoids		
marijuana	cannabis sativa (leaves, flowers)	grass, hay, joints, Mary Jane, pot, reefer, rope, smoke, weed
hashish	cannabis sativa, resin	hash
Volatile Solvents and Gases		
benzine	gasoline	
toluol	glue vapor	
carbon tetrachloride	cleaning fluid	scrubwoman's kick
naphtha	cleaning fluid	
amyl nitrite	amyl nitrite	amys, pears, snapper, poppers
nitrous oxide	nitrous oxide	laughing gas, nitrous

*Many of these drugs are sold under a variety of trade names; only a single popular example is used for each.

TABLE OF DRUGS USED IN PSYCHIATRY

Generic Names

Trade Names
(Examples)

ANTIANXIETY DRUGS

Antihistamine Derivatives
hydroxyzine — Atarax, Vistaril

Benzodiazepine Derivatives
alprazolam — Xanax
chlordiazepoxide — Ampoxide, Librium, Libritabs, Sk-lygen
clonazepam — Klonopin
clorazepate — Tranxene
diazepam — Valium
halazepam — Paxipam
lorazepam — Ativan
oxazepam — Serax
prazepam — Centrax

Non-benzodiazepine
buspirone — BuSpar

ANTIDEPRESSANT DRUGS

Hydrazine MAO Inhibitors
isocarboxazid — Marplan
phenelzine — Nardil

Non-hydrazine MAO Inhibitors
tranylcypromine — Parnate

Generic Names	Trade Names (Examples)
Tricyclic Derivatives	
amitriptyline	Amitril, Elavil, Endep
amoxapine	Asendin
desipramine	Norpramin, Pertofrane
doxepin	Adapin, Curetin, Sinequan
imipramine	Imavate, Janimine, Presamine, SK-Pramine, Tofranil
nortriptyline	Aventyl, Pamelor
protriptyline	Vivactil
trimipramine	Surmontil
Atypical Agents	
trazodone	Desyrel

ANTIMANIC DRUGS

lithium carbonate or citrate	Cibalith, Eskalith, Lithane, Lithobid, Lithonate, Lithotabs
carbamazepine	Tegretol
valproate	Depakene

ANTIPSYCHOTIC DRUGS

Butyrophenones	
haloperidol	Haldol
droperidol	Inapsine
Dibenzoxazepines	
loxapine	Daxolin, Loxitane
Dihydroindolones	
molindone	Lidone, Moban

Diphenylbutylpiperidine
pimozide — Orap

Phenothiazine Derivatives

Aliphatic
chlorpromazine — Thorazine
triflupromazine — Vesprin

Piperazine
acetophenazine — Tindal
butaperazine — Repoise
carphenazine — Proketazine
fluphenazine — Prolixin, Permitil
perphenazine — Trilafon
trifluoperazine — Stelazine

Piperidine
mesoridazine — Serentil
piperacetazine — Quide
thioridazine — Mellaril

Thioxanthene Derivatives
chlorprothixene — Taractan
thiothixene — Navane

TABLE OF LEGAL TERMS

care and protection proceedings Intervention by a court on behalf of a child's health, education, and welfare when the parents or caretakers are unwilling or unable to provide them.

competency to stand criminal trial The test for competency to stand criminal trial applies to the defendant's state of mind at the time of the trial. A person is competent to stand trial when (1) he understands the nature of the charge he faces and the consequences that may result from his conviction, and (2) he is able to rationally assist his attorney in his defense.

conservatorship In most jurisdictions this status means that the conservatee is under the control of another person or persons (conservator) with respect to fiscal or contractual affairs but not with respect to the physical person or body (as with consent to medical or surgical treatment).

criminal responsibility A defendant's state of mind at the time of the alleged crime. A person cannot be convicted of a crime if it can be proved that he lacked the ability to formulate a criminal intent at the time of the alleged crime because of "criminal insanity." See *insanity defense*.

emancipated minor A minor who can be considered to have the rights of an adult when it can be shown that he is, in fact, exercising general control over his life.

expert witness A status conferred on a witness based on appropriate qualifications, training, and experience which acknowledges that competence and authority of the witness in a particular area of expertise. Expert witnesses are permitted to offer opinions in court related to their area of expertise which would not be permitted a witness without such status.

Gault decision A landmark case which states that juvenile court proceedings must measure up to the essentials of due process and fair treatment under the l4th amendment. Namely, the juvenile must be (1) given proper notice of the charges, (2) represented by counsel, (3) protected against self-incrimination, and (4) able to confront and cross-examine witnesses.

guardianship In most jurisdictions, in the context of mental illness, a person under guardianship by reason of mental illness is under the total control of another person or persons and in the status of a ward with respect to both his body (as in consenting to surgery) and fiscal or contractual affairs.

habeas corpus The legal term most commonly used to describe a petition which asks a court to decide whether confinement, of any sort, has been accomplished without due process of law.

incompetency Although this term is often used globally to denote lack of capacity to legally consent or to make a contract, in fact, there are many more specific competencies with their own particular required elements. (See the definitions of *competency to stand criminal trial*, *informed consent*, and *testamentary capacity* elsewhere in this table with their particular required elements.)

informed consent Permission to perform a medical or research procedure which includes: (1) a rational understanding of the nature of the proceedings; (2) the foreseeable risks; (3) the expected benefits; (4) the consequences of withholding consent; (5) available alternative procedures; and (6) that consent is voluntary.

insanity defense A legal concept that a person cannot be convicted of a crime if he lacked *criminal responsibility* by reason of insanity, which term is defined as a matter of law. The premise is that where an alleged criminal lacks the *mens rea* because of insanity, such a person lacks criminal responsibility and cannot be convicted. Standards which the courts in Anglo-American law have established to define insanity have changed over the last century and continue to change. The major landmark decisions defining insanity are:

M'Naghten Rule The English House of Lords in 1843 ruled that a person was not responsible for a crime if the accused "was laboring under such a defect of reason from disease of the mind as not to know the nature and quality of the act; or, if he did know it, that he did not know that what he was doing was wrong." This rule still obtains in most states.

irresistible impulse test The rule that a person is not responsible for a crime if he acts through an irresistible impulse which he was unable to control because of a mental disease. Still accepted in some states, but rejected by most. Introduced in 1922.

Durham Rule A ruling by the U.S. Court of Appeals for the District of Columbia in 1954 that held that "an accused is not criminally responsible if his unlawful act was the product of mental disease or mental defect." Since replaced in the District of Columbia by the *American Law Institute Formulation* (see following).

American Law Institute Formulation Section 4.01 of the ALI's Model Penal Code states that "a person is not responsible for criminal conduct if at the time of such conduct as a result of mental disease or defect he lacks the substantial capacity either to appreciate the wrongfulness of his conduct or to conform his conduct to the requirements of law." Adopted by the Second Circuit U.S. Court of Appeals in 1966 and by the U.S. Court of Appeals for the District of Columbia in 1972 (United States *vs* Brawner).

mens rea An intent to do harm. In a criminal case involving a defendant's mental state, an important question may be whether or not he had mens rea, the ability to form an intention to do harm.

parens patriae In the context of mental illness, this term refers to the constitutional power of the state to involuntarily commit those mentally ill persons who are in need of care and treatment for their mental illness.

police power In the context of mental illness, this term refers to the constitutional power of the state to involuntarily commit mentally ill persons in order to prevent harm (usually physical harm) to the self or other.

privilege The legal right of a patient, always established by statute, to prevent his physician from testifying about information obtained in the course of his treatment by the physician. Thus, a legal affirmation of the ethical principle of *confidentiality*. See *privileged communication* following.

privileged communication The laws of evidence in some jurisdictions provide that certain kinds of communications between persons who have a special confidential or fiduciary relationship will not be divulged. The psychotherapist-patient and doctor-patient relationship is, in some states, considered privileged communication. But the law is in a state of flux and there are many exceptions—e.g., a patient who sues, basing the suit in whole or in part on psychiatric considerations, may waive privilege. It is important to realize that the privilege belongs to the patient not to the therapist, and can be waived only by the patient unless otherwise provided by the law in legal proceedings.

right to refuse treatment Legal doctrine holding that a person, even when involuntarily committed to a hospital, may not be forced to submit to any form of treatment against his will unless a life and death emergency exists.

right to treatment The legal doctrine that a facility is legally obligated to provide adequate treatment for an individual when the facility has assumed the responsibility of providing treatment.

testamentary capacity In the executing of a legally valid will, the basic required legal elements are: (a) the approximate monetary value and nature of the estate should be known by the testator; (b) he should know the natural heirs to his bounty (that is, a spouse or other blood related persons to whom the estate would ordinarily be expected to go); (c) he should know that the instrument (will) that he is signing is, in fact, a will; and (d) he should know the beneficiaries of the will.

TABLE OF NEUROLOGIC DEFICITS

abulia A reduction in impulse to action and thought coupled with indifference or lack of concern about the consequences of action.

acalculia Loss of previously possessed facility with arithmetic calculation.

adiadochokinesia Inability to perform rapid alternating movements of one or more of the extremities.

agnosis Inability to recognize objects presented by way of one or more sensory modalities that cannot be explained by a defect in elementary sensation or a reduced level of consciousness or alertness.

spatial agnosis Inability to recognize spatial relations; disordered spatial orientation.

agraphia Loss of a previously possessed facility for writing.

akathisia A state of motor restlessness ranging from a feeling of inner disquiet to inability to sit still or lie quietly.

akinetic mutism A state of apparent alertness with following eye movements but no speech or voluntary motor responses.

alexia Loss of a previously possessed reading facility that cannot be explained by defective visual acuity.

anosognosia The apparent unawareness of or failure of recognition of one's own functional defect; e.g., hemiplegia, hemianopia.

aphasia Loss of a previously possessed facility of language comprehension or production which cannot be explained by sensory or motor defects or diffuse cerebral dysfunction.

anomic or amnestic aphasia Loss of the ability to name objects.

Broca's aphasia Loss of the ability to product spoken and (usually) written language with comprehension retained.

Wernicke's aphasia Loss of the ability to comprehend language, coupled with production of inappropriate language.

apraxia Loss of a previously possessed ability to perform skilled motor acts which cannot be explained by weakness, abnormal muscle tone or elementary incoordination.

constructional apraxia An acquired difficulty in drawing two-dimensional objects or forms, or in producing or copying three-dimensional arrangements of forms or shapes.

astereognosis Inability to recognize familiar objects by touch that cannot be explained by a defect of elementary tactile sensation.

ataxia Failure of muscle coordination; irregularity of muscle action.

autotopagnosia Inability to localize and name the parts of one's own body.

finger agnosia Autotopagnosia restricted to the fingers.

confabulation Fabrication of stories in response to questions about situations or events that are not recalled.

dys- Prefix usually used to indicate that a function has never developed normally; thus **dyscalculia**, **dysgraphia**, **dyslexia**, dysphasia, and dyspraxia. The prefix may also be used to indicate a perversion of normal function or an incomplete defect.

dysarthria Difficulty in speech production due to incoordination of speech apparatus.

dysgeusia Perversion of the sense of taste.

echolalia Parrot-like repetition of overheard words or fragments of speech.

gegenhalten "Active" resistance to passive movement of the extremities which does not appear to be under voluntary control.

perseveration Tendency to emit the same verbal or motor response again and again to varied stimuli.

prosopagnosia Inability to recognize familiar faces not explained by defective visual acuity or reduced consciousness or alertness.

sensory extinction Failure to report sensory stimuli from one region if another region is stimulated simultaneously, even though when the region in question is stimulated by itself, the stimulus is correctly reported.

simultanagnosia Inability to comprehend more than one element of a visual scene at the same time or to integrate the parts into a whole.

TABLE OF PSYCHOLOGIC TESTS

Test	Type	Assesses	Age of Patient	Output	Administration
Bayley Scales of Infant Development	Infant development	Cognitive functioning and motor development	1-30 months	Performance on subtests measuring cognitive and motor development	Individual
Bender Visual-Motor Gestalt Test	Projective visual-motor development	Personality conflicts Ego function and structure Organic brain damage	5-Adult	Patient's reproduction of geometric figures	Indiviudal
Benton Visual Retention Test	Objective performance	Organic brain damage	Adult	Patient's reproduction of geometric figures from memory	Individual
Cattell Infant Intelligence Scale	Infant development	General motor and cognitive development	1-18 months	Performance on developmental tasks	Individual
Children's Apperception Test (CAT)	Projective	Personality conflicts	Child	Patient makes up stories after viewing pictures	Individual

Test	Type	Assesses	Age of Patient	Output	Administration
Draw-A-Person Draw-A-Family House-Tree	Projective	Personality conflicts Self-image (DAF) Family perception (DAF) Ego functions Intellectual functioning (DAP) Visual-motor coordination	2-Adult	Patient's drawings on a blank sheet of paper	Individual
Frostig Developmental Test of Visual Perception	Visual perception	Eye-motor coordination Figure ground perception Constancy of shape Position in space Spatial relationships	4-8 years	Performance on paper and pencil test measuring five aspects of visual perception	Individual or group
Gesell Developmental Schedules	Preschool development	Cognitive, motor, language and social development	1-60 months	Performance on developmental tasks	Individual
Halstead-Reitan Neuropsychological Battery and Other Measures	Brain functioning	Cerebal functioning and organic brain damage	6-Adult	Various subtests measure aspects of cerebral functioning	Individual

Test					
Illinois Test of Psycholinguistic Ability (ITPA)	Language ability	Auditory-vocal, visual-motor channels of language; receptive, organizational, and expressive components	2-10 years	Performance on 12 sub-tests measuring various dimensions of language functioning	Individual
Michigan Picture Stories	Defensive structure	Personality conflicts	Adolescent	Patient makes up stories after viewing stimulus pictures	Individual
Minnesota Multiphasic Personality Inventory (MMPI)	Paper and pencil; personality inventory	Personality structure Diagnostic classification	Adolescent-Adult	Personality profile reflecting nine dimensions of personality Diagnosis based upon actuarial prediction	Group
Otis Quick Scoring Mental Abilities Tests	Intelligence	Intellectual functioning	5-Adult	Performance on verbal and nonverbal dimensions of intellectual functioning	Group

Test	Type	Assesses	Age of Patient	Output	Administration
Rorschach	Projective	Personality conflicts Ego function and structure Defensive structure Thought processes Affective integration	3-Adult	Patient's associations to inkblots	Individual
Senior Apperception Test (SAT)	Projective	Personality conflicts	Over 65	Patient makes up stories after viewing stimulus pictures	Individual
Stanford-Binet	Intelligence	Intellectual functioning	2-Adult	Performance on problem solving and developmental tasks	Individual
Tasks of Emotional Development (TED)	Projective	Personality conflicts	Child and Adolescent	Patient makes up stories after viewing stimulus pictures	Individual
Thematic Apperception Test (TAT)	Projective	Personality conflicts	Adult	Patient makes up stories after viewing stimulus pictures	Individual

Vineland Social Maturity Scale	Social maturity	Capacity for independent functioning	0-25 + years	Performance on developmental tasks measuring various dimensions of social functioning	Interview patient or guardian of patient, occasional self-report
Wechsler Adult Intelligence Scale (WAIS)	Intelligence	Intellectual functioning	16-Adult	Performance on 10 sub-tests measuring various dimensions of intellectual functioning	Individual
Wechsler Intelligence Scale for Children (WISC)	Intelligence	Intellectual functioning, Thought processes, Ego functioning	5-15	See above	Individual
Wechsler Preschool Primary Scale of Intelligence (WPPSI)	Intelligence	Intellectual functioning, Thought processes, Ego functioning	4-6½ years	See above	Individual

TABLE OF RESEARCH TERMS

analysis of variance (ANOVA) A widely used statistical procedure for determining the significance of differences obtained on an experimental variable studied under two or more conditions. Differences are commonly assigned to three aspects: the individual differences among the subjects or patients studied, group differences, however classified (e.g., by sex), and differences according to the various treatments to which they have been assigned. The method can assess both the main effects of a variable and its interaction with other variables that have been studied simultaneously.

attributable risk The rate of the disorder in exposed subjects that can be attributed to the exposure derived from subtracting the rate (usually **incidence** or mortality) of the disorder of the nonexposed population from the corresponding rate of the exposed population.

concordance In genetic studies, the similarity in a twin pair with respect to the presence or absence of a disease or trait.

control The term is used in three contexts: (1) the process of keeping the relevant conditions of an experiment constant, (2) causing an **independent variable** to vary in a specified and known manner, and (3) using a spontaneously occurring and discoverable fact as a check or standard of comparison to evaluate the facts obtained after the manipulation of the independent variable.

control group In the ideal case, a group of subjects matched as closely as possible to an experimental group of subjects on all relevant aspects and exposed to the same treatments except the independent variable under investigation.

correlation The extent to which two measures vary together, or a measure of the strength of the relationship between two variables. It is usually expressed by a coefficient which varies between +1.0, perfect agreement, and −1.0, a perfect inverse relationship. A correlation coefficient of 0.0 would mean a perfectly random relationship. The correlation coefficient signifies the degree to which knowledge of one score or variable can predict the score on the other variable. A high correlation between two variables does not necessarily indicate a causal relationship between them: the correlation may follow because each of the variables is highly related to a third yet unmeasured factor.

criterion variable Something to be predicted.

demand characteristics The sum total of cues (derived from the manner in which the subject is solicited, the manner in which he is treated by the experimenter, the scuttlebutt about the experiment, the experimental instructions, and, most important, the experimental procedure itself) that communicates the purpose of the experiment and the nature of the behavior expected of the subject. Subjects may confirm the investigator's hypothesis in an effort to behave appropriately rather than responding directly to the independent variables under investigation. By extension, as applied to nonexperimental settings, the tendency of individuals to live up to what is implicitly expected of them, a factor that may play a major role in the outcome of treatment.

discordance In genetic studies, dissimilarity in a twin pair with respect to the presence or absence of a disease or trait.

double-blind A study in which a number of treatments, usually one or more drugs and a placebo, are compared in such a way that neither the patient nor the persons directly involved in the treatment know which preparation is being administered.

ecological validity The extent to which controlled experimental results can be generalized beyond the confines of the particular experimental context of a variety of contexts in the real world.

experimental design The logical framework of an experiment which maximizes the probability of obtaining or detecting real effects and minimizes the likelihood of ambiguities regarding the significance of the experimentally observed differences.

experimental study designs
    case control An investigation in which groups of individuals are selected in terms of whether they do (cases) or do not (controls) have the disorder, the etiology of which is being studied.

cohort An important form of epidemiologic investigation to test hypotheses regarding the causation of disease. The distinguishing factors are: (1) the group or groups of persons to be studied (the cohorts) are defined in terms of characteristics evident prior to appearance of the disorder being investigated; (2) the study groups so defined are observed over a period of time to determine the frequency of the disorder among them.

cross sectional Study in which measurements are made in different samples at the same point in time.

independent group Different treatments are given to different groups; for example, comparing an untreated group with a treated group. Methodologically very sound, but often requires large samples if there is much variability between individuals.

longitudinal Study in which observations on the same individuals are made at two or more different points in time. Most cohort and **case-control** studies are longitudinal.

prospective Study based on data or events which occur subsequent in time relative to the initiation of the investigation. This type of predictive study usually requires many years in order to develop a large enough study population.

retrospective Study based on data or events that occurred prior in time relative to the investigation.

subjects as their own control The same individual is compared with himself before and after a given treatment. This has the advantage of decreasing error variance and the likelihood of showing significant differences with relatively small groups, though it has the disadvantage of practice effects that may occur with repeated measurements.

experimenter bias Experimenter expectations that are inadvertently communicated to patients or subjects. Such expectations may influence experimental findings.

external validity The applicability of the generalizations that may be made from the experimental findings beyond the occasion with those specific subjects, experimental conditions, experimenters, or measurements.

falsifiable hypothesis A hypothesis stated in sufficiently precise fashion that it can be tested by acceptable rules of logic, empirical and statistical evidence, and thereby found to be either confirmed or disconfirmed. An unfalsifiable hypothesis is one that is so general and/or ambiguous that all conceivable evidence can be "explained" by it.

heuristic Serving to encourage discovery of problem solutions.

incidence The number of cases of disease which come into being during a specific period of time.

intervening variable Something intervening between an antecedent circumstance and its consequence, modifying the relation between the two. For example, appetite can be an intervening variable determining whether or not a given food will be eaten. The intervening variable may be inferred rather than empirically detected.

mean The arithmetic average of a set of observations; the sum of scores divided by the number of scores.

median The middle value in a set of values that have been arranged in order from highest to lowest.

mode The most frequently occurring observation in a set of observations.

non-parametric tests of significance When data do not satisfy certain statistical assumptions, such as being normally distributed, other specialized statistical procedures which do not require assumptions of normality must be employed. These methods are often based upon an analysis of ranks rather than on the distribution of the actual scores themselves. Widely used examples are the chi-square, Spearman rank order correlation, median, and Mann-Whitney U tests.

null hypothesis Testing the null hypothesis requires a computation to determine the limits within which two groups may differ in their results (e.g., an **experimental** and a **control group**— even though if the experiment were often repeated or the groups were larger no difference would be found. The probability of the obtained difference being found if no true difference existed is commonly expressed as a p-value, e.g., $p < .05$ that the null hypothesis is true.

operational definition The meaning of a concept when it is translated into terms amenable to systematic observation and measurement, e.g., temperature defined by a thermometer reading under standard conditions.

parameter Any quantitative value that a variable can take.

parametric study One which examines the effects on **a dependent variable** of variations, usually across a broad range, in the values of the **independent variable.**

parametric tests of significance Tests based on the assumption that the form of the distribution of the observations is known, usually a so-called normal distribution. Widely used tests based on such as assumption include analysis of variance, t-tests, and Pearsonian correlation coefficients.

period prevalence A measure that expresses the total number of cases of a disease known to have existed at some time during a specified period. It is the sum of **point prevalence** and **incidence.**

placebo In psychopharmacology, a pill which contains no pharmacologically active ingredient.

active placebo The presence or absence of side effects may allow the patient to identify whether he is receiving drug or placebo (for example, dry mouth may be associated with chlorpromazine). An active placebo is one which may mimic the side effects, but does not have the specific and assumed therapeutic pharmacologic action of the drug under investigation.

placebo effect Either therapeutic effects or side effects following the ingestion of a placebo. By extension, one may speak of a placebo effect as the non-specific aspects of any treatment procedure, usually mediated by the patient's expectations of improvement, such as the placebo effect of psychotherapy.

point prevalence The frequency of the disease at a designated point in time.

population A statistical concept that refers to all individuals or instances that theoretically could be available for study or measurement. Statistical inference involves generalizing from the observation of some specified sample to the population.

practice effects The modification in task performances as a result of repeated trials or training in the task.

predictor variable The test or other form of performance which is used to predict the person's status on a **criterion variable**. For example, scores on the Scholastic Aptitude Test might be used to predict the criterion "finishing college within the top 33% of graduating class." Scores on the Scholastic Aptitude Test would be predictor scores.

quantitative variable An object of observation which varies in manner or degree in such a way that it may be measured.

q-sort A personality assessment technique in which the subject (or someone who observes him) indicates the degree to which a standardized set of descriptive statements actually describes the subject. The term reflects the "sorting" procedures occasionally used with this technique.

random sample A group of subjects selected in such a way that each member of the population from which the sample is derived has an equal or known chance (probability) of being chosen for the sample.

relative risk The ratio of the disorder (usually **incidence** of mortality) of those exposed to the rate of those not exposed.

reliability The extent to which the same test or procedure will yield the same result either over time or with different observers. The most commonly reported reliabilities are (1) test-retest reliability—the correlation between the first and second test of a number of subjects; (2) the split-half reliability—the correlation within a single test of two similar parts of the test; and (3) inter-rater reliability—the agreement between different individuals scoring the same procedure or observations.

selection bias The inadvertent selection of a non-representative sample of subjects or observations. A classic example is a 1936 Literary Digest poll which predicted Landon's election over Roosevelt because telephone directories were used as basis for selecting respondents.

significance level The arbitrarily selected probability level for rejecting the **null hypothesis**, commonly .05 or .01.

significant differences When statistical tests show that a given difference is not likely to have occurred by chance. In many behavioral studies, the likelihood of an event occurring less frequently than 1 in 20 times ($p < .05$) is considered the minimal acceptable significance level. The determination that a given difference between two groups is significant can merely serve to identify the likelihood that it was not a chance event. In no way does this prove that the demonstrated systematic difference is necessarily due to the reasons hypothesized by an investigator. Systematic factors not considered by the investigator can sometimes be responsible for significant differences.

standard deviation (SD) A mathematical measure of the dispersion or spread of scores clustered about the **mean**. In any distribution which approximates the normal curve in form, about 65% of the measurements will lie within one SD of the mean, and about 95% will lie within two SDs of the mean.

statistical inference The process of using a limited sample of data to infer something about a larger population of potentially obtainable data which has not been observed.

test of significance A comparison of the observed probability of an event with the predicted probability which is based on calculations deduced from statistical chance distributions of such events.

type I error The error which is made when the **null hypothesis** is true, but as the result of the **test of significance** is rejected or declared false.

type II error The error which is made when the **null hypothesis** is false, but due to the results of the **test of significance** is not rejected or declared false.

theory A general statement predicting, explaining, or describing the relationships among a number of constructs.

variable Any characteristic in an experiment which may assume different values.

   independent variable The variable under the experimenter's control.

dependent variable That aspect of the subject which is measured after the manipulation of the **independent variable** and assumed to vary as a function of the independent variable.

variance The square of the **standard deviation**. Used in analysis of variance.

volunteer bias Individuals who volunteer for some procedures are not generally representative of the total population. Self-selected patients who seek out treatment based upon newspaper publicity, for example, are likely to do significantly better than random patients who are simply offered the treatment.

zygosity (1) *dizygotic*: fraternal twins, the product of two fertilized ova. They have the genetic relationship of any two siblings; (2) *monozygotic*: identical twins, the product of a single fertilized ovum.

TABLE OF SCHOOLS OF PSYCHIATRY

I. Reconstructive

  A. Psychoanalysis—Sigmund **Freud**

  B. Neo-Freudian, modifications of psychoanalysis
    1. Active analytic techniques—Sandor Ferenczi, Wilheim Stekel, the Chicago school (especial Franz **Alexander** and Thomas French)
    2. Analytic play therapy—Anna **Freud**, Melanie **Klein**
    3. Analytic psychology—Carl **Jung**
    4. Character analysis, orgone therapy—Wilheim **Reich**
    5. Cognitive—Jean **Piaget**
    6. Developmental—Erik **Erikson**
    7. Ego psychology—Paul Federn, Eduardo Weiss, Heinz Hartmann, Ernst Kris, Rudolph Loewenstein
    8. Existential analysis—Ludwig Binswanger
    9. Holistic analysis—Karen **Horney**
    10. Individual psychology—Alfred **Adler**
    11. Transactional analysis—Eric Berne
    12. Washington cultural school—Harry Stack **Sullivan**, Erich Fromm, Clara Thompson
    13. Will therapy—Otto **Rank**

  C. Group Approaches
    1. Orthodox psychoanalytic—S.R. Slavson
    2. Psychodrama—Jacob L. Moreno
    3. Psychoanalysis in groups—Alexander Wolf
    4. Valence systems—Walter Bion

II. Reeducative and Supportive, Individual and Group
    1. Client-centered (non-directive)—Carl **Rogers**
    2. Conditioning, behavior therapy, behavior modification
      a. aversion therapy—N.V. Kantorovich
      b. behaviorism—John B. **Watson**
      c. classical conditioning—Ivan **Pavlov**
      d. operant conditioning—Burrhus F. **Skinner**
      e. sexual counseling—William Masters, Virginia Johnson

    f. systematic desensitization—Joseph Wolpe
3. Cognitive behavior—Aaron Beck
4. Family therapy—Nathan Ackerman
5. Gestalt—Wolfgang, Kohler, Kurt Lewin, Fritz Perls
6. Logotherapy—Victor Frankl
7. Psychobiology (distributive analysis and synthesis)—Adolf **Meyer**
8. Zen (satori)—Alan Watts